D1214411

Special Care Dentistry

Quintessentials of Dental Practice – 42
Clinical Practice – 5

Special Care Dentistry

By

Janice Fiske
Chris Dickinson
Carole Boyle
Sobia Rafique
Mary Burke

Editor-in-Chief: Nairn H F Wilson
Editor Clinical Practice: Nairn H F Wilson

Quintessence Publishing Co. Ltd.
London, Berlin, Chicago, Paris, Milan, Barcelona, Istanbul,
São Paulo, Tokyo, New Delhi, Moscow, Prague, Warsaw

British Library Cataloguing in Publication Data

Special care dentistry. - (Quintessentials of dental practice; v. 42)
  1. People with disabilities - Dental care 2. Dentistry - Practice
  I. Fiske, Janice II. Wilson, Nairn H. F.
  617.6'0087

ISBN-13: 9781850971344

Copyright © 2007 Quintessence Publishing Co. Ltd., London

All rights reserved. This book or any part thereof may not be reproduced, stored in a retrieval system, or transmitted in any form or by any means, electronic, mechanical, photocopying, or otherwise, without the written permission of the publisher.

ISBN-13: 978-1-85097-134-4

Foreword

Special Care Dentistry is special on many counts. Patients requiring Special Care Dentistry pose special challenges; special skills and knowledge are integral to successful clinical outcomes, and special care and attention is fundamental to the planning and effective delivery of care.

This book is timely, given the growing need and demand for Special Care Dentistry around the world. Advances in healthcare, people living longer, and attitudinal changes in society are but three of the many, varied reasons for the growth and increasing practice of Special Care Dentistry.

In the provision of oral healthcare to individuals with disabilities, disorders and other conditions falling within the scope of Special Care Dentistry, the most appropriate and effective treatment may be relatively straightforward and minimally interventive – indeed, often the simpler the better, but the management of the patient tends to be complex and challenging. Understanding and dealing with these complexities and challenges is the focus of this excellent addition to the highly successful, wide-ranging *Quintessentials of Dental Practice* series: comprehensive, yet succinct; authoritative, but pragmatic; and of immediate clinical relevance, rather than theoretical. To add to these qualities, this book is most engaging and easy to read, given the carefully crafted text, supported by numerous high-quality illustrations.

Practitioners, let alone students, and even those with special interests in the field will extend and enhance their understanding and appreciation of Special Care Dentistry in the few hours it takes to read this book from cover to cover – an enjoyable, thought-provoking and informative experience. And once read, this book will become a trusted reference text to turn to for practical guidance and situation-saving clinical tips. All in all, another gem in the bejewelled *Quintessentials'* crown.

Nairn Wilson
Editor-in-Chief

Contents

Chapter 1
Understanding Special Care Dentistry

Aim

The aim of this chapter is to explain what is meant by Special Care Dentistry, who requires it, why he or she requires it and who can provide it.

Outcome

After reading this chapter you should have an understanding of what is meant by Special Care Dentistry and the part that you can play in its delivery.

Introduction

The main purpose of this book is twofold:
• Firstly to remove the stereotypes and myths that can surround people who require Special Care Dentistry, and
• Secondly to provide the dental team with knowledge, information and practical tips that will encourage them to undertake Special Care Dentistry.

What is Special Care Dentistry?

Special Care Dentistry is concerned with providing and enabling the delivery of oral care for people with an impairment or disability, where this terminology is defined in the broadest of terms. Thus, Special Care Dentistry is concerned with: *The improvement of oral health of individuals and groups in society who have a physical, sensory, intellectual, mental, medical, emotional or social impairment or disability or, more often, a combination of a number of these factors.*

It is defined by a diverse client group with a range of disabilities and complex additional needs and includes people living at home, in long-stay residential care and secure units, as well as homeless people. Clearly, not every individual encompassed by this definition requires specialist care and the majority of people can, and should, be treated by the primary dental care network of general, personal and salaried dental services.

The Ethos of Special Care Dentistry

The ethos of Special Care Dentistry is its broad-based philosophy of provision of care. It achieves the greatest benefit for patients by taking a holistic view of oral health, and liaising and working with all those members of an individual's care team (be they dental, medical or social) to achieve the most appropriate care plan and treatment for that person through an integrated care pathway.

Special Care Dentistry is proactive to the needs of people with disabilities rather than solely reactive. Recognising that some groups of people are unable to access oral healthcare unaided, to express a desire or need for oral healthcare or to make an informed decision about its benefits to them, Special Care Dentistry includes screening, preventive, and treatment programmes tailored to meet the specific needs of groups or individuals.

Its guiding principles are that:
• All individuals have a right to equal standards of health and care.
• All individuals have a right to autonomy, as far as possible, in relation to decisions made about them.
• Good oral health has positive benefits for health, dignity and self-esteem, social integration, and general nutrition and the impact of poor oral health can be profound.

Definition of Disability

Disability is difficult to define. Words mean different things to different people. While some people prefer to be referred to as "disabled people" (as it clarifies that their disability is related to society's barriers), others prefer to be called "people with disabilities" (emphasising that they are people first and disabled second). However, there are also cultural differences in the use of terminology. For example, as Nunn points out, in African languages there are words to describe observable impairments like lameness but no overarching generic terms. Some cultures consider names as stigmatising, and in the UK the terminology "mental retardation" is considered to be stigmatising and unacceptable, whereas in the USA it is considered acceptable and is a currently used term.

The language of disability can be confusing. It is continually changing, reflecting developments in legislation and understanding of the complex issues surrounding it. Whilst there are different causes and different types of disability it is important to remember that everyone with a disability is an individual with their own set of needs and wants.

In the UK, terms in general use are impairment and disability, where:
- ***Impairment*** refers to a medical condition or malfunction
- ***Disability*** refers to the restrictions caused by society through discrimination, ignorance or prejudice.

Within this book, the term disability will be used to refer to all those people who require Special Care Dentistry, including those with complex medical conditions.

Demography of Disability – One in Four of Us

It is estimated that between 8.6 and 10.8 million people in Great Britain are disabled (see Table 1-1) and that the life of one in every four adults in the UK will be affected by disability, either through experiencing a disability or caring for someone close to them who has a disability.

The number of people with a long-term illness, health problem, or disability which limits their daily activities or work increased significantly

Table 1-1 **Incidence of disability**

Types of impairment	Estimated numbers affected
Visual impairments	2 million
Hearing impairments	8.7 million
Mobility impairments (wheelchair users)	500,000
Learning difficulties	1 million
Invisible or "hidden" impairments	250,000
Arthritis	8 million
Mental health impairments	1 in 4 of the population

between the 1991 and 2001 surveys. Census data for England and Wales indicate that almost 9.5 million people (18.2% of the population) self-report a long-term illness, health problem, or disability which limits their daily activities or work. Disability tends to increase with age and multiple disabilities are more likely to occur in old age with approximately two-thirds of all people with a disability being over 65 years of age. The prevalence and common causes of disability for the different age groups are shown in Table 1-2.

There is no single register for disability, and a proportion of people with disability have multiple impairments and/or medical conditions so that the categories of disability and impairment may overlap. For example, people with learning impairments have an increased prevalence of associated disabilities such as physical or sensory impairments, behavioural differences and epilepsy. Furthermore, with ageing, people with learning disabilities also have a higher rate of dementia than the general population.

Table 1-2 **Age, prevalence and common causes of disability**

Age group	Prevalence of disability	Common causes of disability
< 16 years	4.3%	1. Genetic and congenital disorders
16–49 years	9.65%	1. Trauma (e.g. spinal and head injuries) 2. Neurological (e.g. multiple sclerosis)
50–64 years	26.6%	1. Musculoskeletal disorders (e.g. osteoarthritis) 2. Cardiorespiratory disorders (e.g. ischaemic heart disease and obstructive airway disease) 3. Neurological disorders (e.g. stroke)
65+ years	51.5%	

The Disability Discrimination Act (DDA) 1995

Within the terms of the UK DDA 1995, a disabled person is defined as someone who has a physical or mental impairment that has a substantial and long-term adverse effect on his or her ability to carry out normal day-to-day activities. The DDA 1995, together with related Codes of Practice, introduced measures aimed at ending discrimination and giving rights to disabled people. It was introduced in phases (see Table 1-3).

Essentially it requires that providers must:
- Take reasonable steps to change policies, practices and procedures which make it unreasonably difficult or impossible for disabled people to use their services.
- Take reasonable steps to remove or alter physical features which could be a barrier to disabled people using their services.
- Provide the service in an alternative way if the removal of such barriers is impossible, for example, where planning consent to adapt a listed building is withheld. In the case of services to people confined to their home, this could mean providing domiciliary dental care.
- Consider access to a service in broad terms that includes access to information about a service. This means that information should be available in alternative formats such as audio, large print formats, etc.

Table 1-3 **The phases and requirements of the DDA 1995**

Phase	Requirement
1. December 1996	It became unlawful for service providers to treat disabled people less favourably for a reason related to their disability
2. October 1999	Providers were required to make reasonable adjustments for disabled people such as providing extra help or making changes to the way they provide their services
3. October 2004	Required service providers to assess obstacles and make reasonable adjustments to the physical features of their premises to overcome physical barriers to access

The Disability Discrimination Act (DDA) 2005

The UK DDA 2005 is designed to extend the rights for disabled people, and clarify and extend the provisions of the DDA 1995. It extends the definition of disability; gives protection against discrimination for people in public service; and creates new legal responsibilities on local authorities, primary care trusts, health authorities and other public bodies to:

- develop and deliver disability equality plans
- demonstrate how they intend to eliminate discrimination and harassment
- promote equal opportunities
- encourage positive attitudes towards disabled people.

The Mental Capacity Act 2007

The UK Mental Capacity Act will be implemented in 2007. It aims to protect people with learning disabilities and mental health conditions, such as Alzheimer's disease. It will provide clear guidelines for carers and professionals about who can take decisions in which situations. The Act states that everyone should be treated as able to take their own decisions until it is shown that they are unable to do so. It aims to enable people to make their own decisions for as long as they are able and a person's ability to make a decision will be established at the time that a decision needs to be made. Additionally, there will be a new criminal offence of neglect or ill-treatment of a person that lacks the capacity.

Current Health and Social Policy

Current health and social policy is focused on the reduction of health inequalities. It recognises that this will not be easy, and that inequalities in health are widening and will continue to do so unless things are done differently through better coordinated activities that cross traditional boundaries so that agencies work in partnership. It particularly refers to improving the quality of life, access to services and addressing healthcare needs for older people, people with mental illness, people with a learning disability, and asylum seekers and refugees. The ethos of Special Care Dentistry echoes this philosophy.

Oral Health and Disability

Disabled people want teeth for the same reasons as other people. They want to look good, feel good about themselves and to be socially acceptable. Additionally, they want their mouths to be comfortable and to be able to enjoy their food. To achieve this end, people increasingly wish to retain their natural teeth.

People with disabilities and complex additional needs should have equal access to oral healthcare services and equitable oral health outcomes in terms of self-esteem, appearance, social interaction, function, and comfort. However, this is not the case. Indeed, whilst people with disability and complex additional needs (particularly those with a learning disability or mental health problems) have similar patterns of oral disease as the general population, they have poorer oral health and poorer health outcomes from care. Lower levels of oral health have been demonstrated in a range of patient groups, including people with cerebral palsy, epilepsy, multiple sclerosis, and psychiatric illness. This situation has also been identified amongst young disabled people, people with learning disabilities, and older people, particularly those in residential care. Furthermore, when oral diseases are treated they are more likely to result in extractions than fillings, crowns and bridges. The British Society for Disability and Oral Health has produced guidelines for oral healthcare and the development of integrated oral healthcare pathways to encourage the move towards equitable access, care and outcomes.

Generally, people requiring Special Care Dentistry have needs which are wider than oral health. For example, providing oral care for persons with a learning disability may involve dealing with their inability to consent for care; the use of tools such as *"Makaton"* and *"Easy Read"*; working with advocates; organising, attending and informing *"Best Interest Meetings"*; and taking responsibility for informed consent.

Dealing with Disabled People

A current, comprehensive medical and social history that is constantly updated is imperative to understanding the needs of all patients including those with disability and complex medical conditions. Not all disabilities are visible and many are "hidden", for example epilepsy, diabetes, positive HIV status and ischaemic heart disease. There is some evidence to show that it is more difficult for people with hidden, than visible, disabilities to ask for the help they need. Also because of the stigma attached to a disability they may not disclose their disability or may even go as far as disguising one disability by pretending that they have another less stigmatising disability; for example, people who cannot read have been known to feign impaired vision.

When meeting a patient with a disability for the first time:
- don't make assumptions – always ask
- be patient – allow time for questions to be answered
- listen – use an active non-judgemental technique

- believe what they tell you
- respect the person for who they are
- gather additional information if required (e.g. from a carer or a healthcare professional)
- when talking to a carer, include the person with the disability in the conversation. Never talk across them, over their heads or about them as if they are not present.

Conclusions

- The majority of people with a disability have disabilities that are mild or moderate and do not require specialist dental care.
- Most people with mild or moderate disability could, and should, receive dental care in mainstream primary dental services.
- This book seeks to encourage you to treat people with disability by providing you and your team with knowledge and information related to Special Care Dentistry.

Further Reading

British Society for Disability and Oral Health's Oral Healthcare Guidelines for various groups of people can be accessed at www.bsdh.org.uk

Nunn J. Disability and Oral Care. London: FDI World Dental Press Ltd, 2000.

The Disability Partnership. One in Four of Us: The Experience of Disability. Accessible at www.disability.org.uk/dp

Chapter 2
Managing the Oral Health of Patients With Physical Disabilities

Aim

The aim of this chapter is to discuss the treatment of those patients who may have difficulties with access to dental care or complying with dental treatment due to physical disability.

Outcome

After reading this chapter you should be able to look at your clinical environment in light of the needs of patients with physical disabilities; and be aware of the requirements and considerations needed when providing oral healthcare outside the dental practice setting.

Introduction

Any significant impairment of function that impacts upon daily life can be viewed as a physical disability; however, it is not synonymous with ill health. The person's disability may be totally separate from health status. For example, Fig 2-1 shows an athlete with an obvious physical impairment that has no impact on health status.

There are many forms of physical disability and this chapter will focus on physical disability relating to motor function. This is usually related to impairments of movement but can also include manual dexterity and speech. This chapter will look at the oral healthcare provision for people with disabilities of movement and dexterity only and discuss issues relating to both the patient and clinician.

Motor function impairments may be attributable to many causes, including:
- congenital deformity – inherited or acquired intrauterine
- acquired impairments – from birth, as in cerebral palsy, or developed during life due to disease process, such as rheumatoid arthritis and any of the chronic neurological disorders

- trauma – due to accidents and incidents
- iatrogenic – as in surgery.

Chronic neurological disorders, such as multiple sclerosis, Parkinson's disease, motor neurone disease and Huntington's disease, tend to be progressive. The rate at which they progress, and the degree of disability that results, can be varied and unpredictable. Their common feature is that medical treatment neither provides a cure nor controls the condition sufficiently to prevent its progression. In the final stages of disease, individuals will require nursing support and palliative care.

The aim of this chapter is to highlight the varied nature of the presentation of motor function impairment rather than discuss all the causes. By way of example, Fig 2-2 shows the hand of a patient with systemic sclerosis (scleroderma) that drastically affects the ability to hold and manipulate a toothbrush. Oral hygiene procedures are severely impaired.

Barriers to Oral Healthcare

Access to oral healthcare facilities is a recognised barrier for people with physical disabilities. The physical and emotional barriers that must be overcome

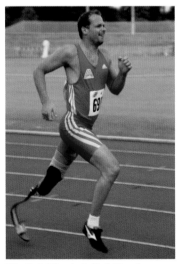

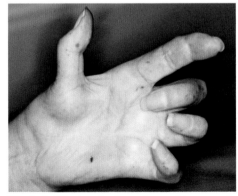

Fig 2-1 Physical disability does not necessarily impact on health status.

Fig 2-2 The hand of a patient with systemic sclerosis (scleroderma).

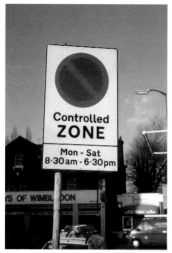

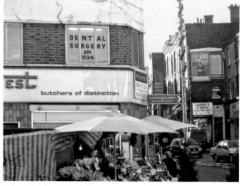

Fig 2-3a Restricted parking. **Fig 2-3b** First-floor surgery in a market area.

in order to attend dental services can be compounded by the cost of treatment as many people with physical disability are on low income. Additionally if carers or assistants are required by the individual this may further complicate matters.

Physical access to dental premises may not be favourable for people with physical disabilities. Stairs, narrow corridors and cramped surgeries may reduce ease of access. Traditional high-street surgery locations may create travel and parking problems as shown in Figs 2-3a and 2-3b.

Stair access to first-floor surgeries may be impossible to negotiate for people with mobility difficulties yet the building may not be amenable to adaptation, for either engineering or financial reasons. Nevertheless, disability discrimination legislation requires every clinician to assess his or her working environment to identify the problem areas and to put practical steps in place to overcome the issues raised. If treatment cannot be provided within the surgery then provision of the service by alternative means is required. This may include domiciliary dentistry or referral to a provider service that can accommodate the patient's needs, possibly through the use of a mobile dental unit.

Additionally, the attitudes and skills of the dental team can be a barrier to care if there is little experience in treating disabled patients.

Improving Access

Ensuring good physical access to your practice is important. The legislation gives disabled people the right to bring a civil claim against your practice if they consider that you have discriminated against them. Damages that can be awarded to the disabled person who has been discriminated against are limitless.

One of the best ways to assess physical access to your practice is to ask for the opinions of people with physical disabilities and/or undertake an access audit. The local authority or one of many commercial companies will be able to help you with this. An approach you might take is set out in Table 2-1.

Access audits identify potential problem areas and recommend solutions across a broad range of issues including:
- the approach to the premises (parking, kerbs, ramps, lighting, etc.)
- the entrance (door width, level threshold, position and design of door handles)
- the reception and waiting room (clear signage, non-slip flooring, communication aids, appropriate seating, space for wheelchairs)

Table 2-1 **An approach to assessing access to the dental practice**

Access to the dental practice	
Assess your practice	Consider what measures you already have in place and how you could improve them
Look for barriers	Ask yourself and your patients, what barriers do physically disabled patients face in this practice?
Ask outsiders/ get advice	Contact the local authority or a commercial company to guide you through complying with the DDA and to provide practical and affordable solutions
Short-term plan	Draw up a 6-month plan with your top priorities and action them
Long-term plan	List longer-term aims over the next 12 months such as staff training, or affordable access improvements

- the corridors (width and space to manoeuvre, no obstructions)
- the surgery (design, and space to manoeuvre)
- toilet facilities (space, transfer bars, raised seat, alarm in place)
- means of escape (visual alarm, exits accessible by all, signage)
- disability awareness training for staff.

Simple changes may improve the access characteristics of the building with minimal outlay. Having made changes, ensure that practice information leaflets explain the facilities. This will increase the awareness among your client group, able bodied and disabled alike. If domiciliary visits are a regular event in the practice it will also explain to patients when and why there is no dentist in attendance at certain times.

Clinical Service Provision

Many patients are independent. Never assume they require assistance to access the dental chair, always ask. Also for some people, such as those with arthritis, being touched is a painful experience. Wheelchair users may be able to transfer from their wheelchair into the dental chair alone. If not, simple transfer devices are available to assist with this task, such as:

- transfer or "banana" boards – smooth-curved boards that can be placed between the seats to allow people to slide from one to the other
- swivel mats – that can be placed on the floor to allow a standing person to rotate to face in another direction without moving their feet. These can be placed on the ground between a wheelchair and dental chair to aid transfer.

Some people with physical disabilities will have difficulty in sitting or reclining in a dental chair and may need to be treated in the semi- or even upright position. This is also necessary for patients with conditions that impair the gag reflex in order to avoid aspiration of saliva, water spray and other dental debris which could result in aspiration pneumonia.

When considering equipment purchase and installation think about its use in all situations, for example:

- can people with physical disability get into this dental chair easily or would a "break-leg" chair be more helpful?
- can this panoramic radiography machine be used for a patient sitting in a chair or wheelchair?
- is the surgery design suitable for wheelchair access?
- is there room for a wheelchair alongside the dental chair – either for easy transfer or to be able to treat the patient in their wheelchair?

- are the storage cupboards or dental chairs located in such a way as to impede access or increase it?
- are doors and corridors wide enough?

Manual Handling Issues

It is not advisable for dental staff to manually transfer patients from their wheelchairs to a dental chair as this can result in damage to the patient (dislocation of shoulders) and to the dental staff (back injury). When patients cannot transfer themselves between wheelchairs and dental chairs, the recommended transfer device is a hoist. Training is required but they allow safe and comfortable transfer.

Once in the dental chair some patients may need assistance to stay comfortable during the visit. Cushions, blankets or pieces of foam can be used to support the head, limbs or body during treatment. If the patient has any uncontrolled limb movements, such as in ataxic cerebral palsy, the limbs may need to be guarded or protected from hitting or knocking against equipment or instruments such as handpieces.

Some patients cannot or should not be transferred from their wheelchair for dental treatment. In this situation, the ultimate device is a wheelchair recliner. There are a number of designs available utilising manual and electric controls. These are expensive but allow the patient to remain in their wheelchair throughout the visit, eliminate transfer risks to both staff and patient, and provide comfort to both the dentist and the patient throughout treatment. A group of dental nurses and dentists undergoing practical training in the use of a fixed wheelchair recliner is shown in Fig 2-4.

Oral Hygiene Aids

Physical disability involving the arms and hands can create difficulties holding toothbrushes and in performing oral hygiene procedures. Electric toothbrushes tend to have larger diameter handles making them easier to grip than most manual brushes but they tend to be heavier and do not suit everyone.

Adapting Toothbrush Handles

There are many different ways of adapting toothbrush handles to improve their grip. The simplest methods involve inserting a toothbrush handle into another material to improve its size, shape or surface characteristics. Sponges, plastazote tubing, bicycle handlebar grips, rubber hose, silicone putty, denture acrylic, and squash, tennis and foam play balls have all been used (Figs 2-5a and 2-5b).

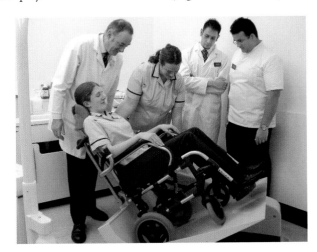

Fig 2-4 Training in the use of a fixed wheelchair recliner.

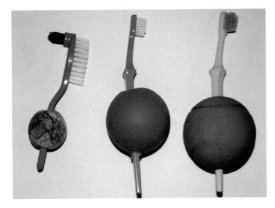

Fig 2-5a Toothbrush handle adaptations using balls.

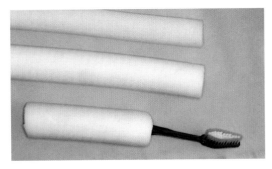

Fig 2-5b Toothbrush handle adaptations using plastazote tubing.

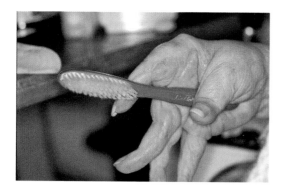

Fig 2-6a Rheumatoid hand.

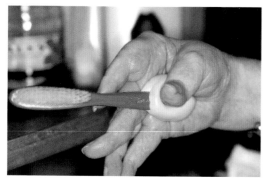

Fig 2-6b Silicone putty "button" to provide grip.

Plastazote tubing and dental silicone putty appear to be the most simple and successful methods. The hand of a patient with severe rheumatoid arthritis is shown in Figs 2-6a and 2-6b. The middle, ring and little fingers of the right hand are non-functional with no joint movement and the grip strength has reduced between the first finger and thumb, making using a denture brush impossible. A silicone putty button was moulded to the patient's denture brush to allow grip between thumb and palm and to prevent the brush from rotating in use. A silicone putty adaptation to a toothbrush handle for a patient with severe Dupuytren's contracture where the ring, middle and little fingers were permanently curled over is shown in Fig 2-6c.

Another technique involves constructing devices to hold the toothbrush/denture brush for the patient. Hand straps can be built with integral sleeves into which toothbrushes can be inserted. Brushes can be bent into a variety of shapes to facilitate cleaning of all areas of the mouth. One such device is shown in use in Figs 2-7a and 2-7b.

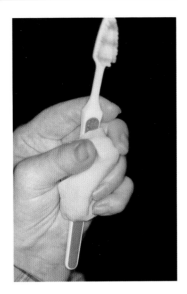

Fig 2-6c Silicone putty addition to provide grip in Dupuytren's contracture.

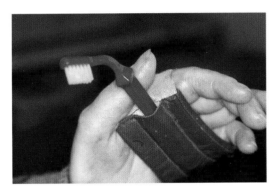

Fig 2-7a Hand strap with integral sleeve to take tooth-brush.

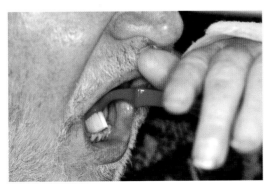

Fig 2-7b Toothbrush bent to provide lingual access to lower incisors.

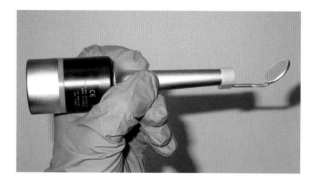

Fig 2-8a Illuminated dental examination mirror.

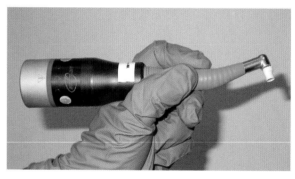

Fig 2-8b Cordless micromotor with prophylaxis handpiece.

Domiciliary Dentistry

People with physical disability who are confined to their homes require domiciliary dental care. Many of these people will be over 65 years of age, a population that increasingly requires restorative dentistry.

Advantages and Disadvantages

Domiciliary dentistry has a number of advantages and disadvantages for both the patient and the dental team. Patients often feel less anxious in their own familiar surroundings, but this also applies to dental staff. What can seem relatively simple in the dental surgery can become difficult and stressful in unfamiliar environments. However, in the home situation you gain more insight into the problems the patient faces regarding compliance with oral healthcare maintenance such as tooth brushing and dietary regimens. In this setting, the dentist may have direct access to other health carers. For example, district nurses can be an invaluable source of help and information; and in care homes the dental team can liaise with the care staff, offering information and advice directly.

Domiciliary visits are time-consuming, not just in the travel to and from the patient's residence, but with the procedures themselves: "set-up" and "clearing-away" time, and traffic and parking issues. Failed appointments are few, but still occur due to patients' competing priorities, such as hospital visits. It is wise to telephone the day before to ensure the visit has not been superseded by something else. Many of the organisational issues relating to domiciliary visits may be carried out by the reception staff or dental nurse. This has a training implication relating, not least importantly, to confidentiality.

The Scope of Domiciliary Dentistry

Traditionally domiciliary dental care was restricted to relatively non-invasive treatments such as denture construction, scaling and simple extractions. If relatively few home visits are undertaken then it is best to keep things straightforward. Simple equipment such as illuminated dental examination mirrors (Fig 2-8a), electric motors for denture adjustment, or micromotors with prophylaxis handpieces (Fig 2-8b) are relatively inexpensive.

With the advent of technologically advanced portable equipment such as the "Minident" (Fig 2-9) and "Dentalman" (Fig 2-10) units, restorative procedures are possible in the domiciliary setting. The functions of domiciliary units vary and can include high and slow speed handpieces, ultrasonic scalers,

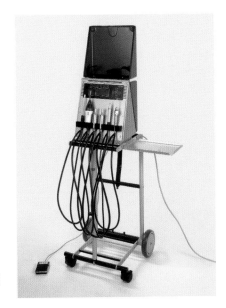

Fig 2-9 "Minident" domiciliary dental unit.

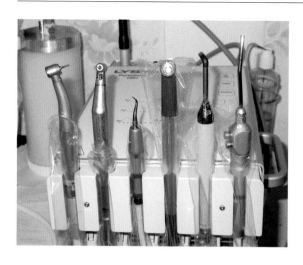

Fig 2-10 "Dentalman" domiciliary dental unit.

three-in-one air and water supply, suction and light curing units. They are expensive, but if large numbers of domiciliary visits are planned then the investment is worthwhile. Lighting can vary from a simple hand-held torch to a dedicated halogen or LED light source. Some of the portable dental units have fibre-optic lights for improved intraoral visibility; optical loupes with integral light sources can also be useful.

One of the most difficult areas of domiciliary dentistry can be the position of the patient for restorative procedures. Domiciliary care is often performed with the clinician standing and the patient seated in a chair that is neither the ideal height nor position for good posture. You must be aware of your, and your nurse's, posture at all times so as not to risk lower back strain.

Planning

Domiciliary treatment requires excellent pretreatment planning skills and good organisational ability. Every piece of equipment required for a procedure will need to be prepared in advance and procedural checklists can help avoid leaving a vital piece of equipment behind. Simple carrying cases, as shown in Fig 2-11, are available and several may be required when contemplating restorative procedures.

People who are restricted to their own homes may present with greater and more severe oral health problems than the general population. Large volumes of treatment and difficult cases may be unsuitable for treatment under domiciliary conditions. In these cases transport to a dental surgery for treat-

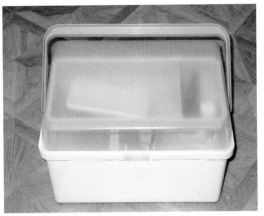

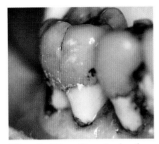

Fig 2-12 Cervical glass ionomer restorations carried out on a domiciliary visit.

Fig 2-11 Domiciliary carrying case.

ment may be the only recourse, or a mix-and-match approach tackling the more complex items of treatment in a surgery setting and the simpler items at home. Simple diagnostic and health education procedures can easily be carried out in a domiciliary setting, as can periodontal probing and scaling. Most full and partial denture construction procedures are also possible in the patient's home.

Restorative care has been revolutionised by the advent of light-cured, adhesive restorations using both glass ionomer and composite materials. Portable curing lights can be used both in and outside the surgery. The use of combined etch, prime and bonding systems reduces the need for separate etching and bonding procedures and rapidly applied rubber dam systems make tooth isolation quick and simple. All are quite feasible in the domiciliary setting. Systems such as those illustrated in Figs 2-9 and 2-10 have fast and slow handpiece capability for cavity preparation with suction and fibre-optic light sources. Cervical root caries lesions restored with glass ionomer cement on a domiciliary basis are shown in Fig 2-12.

Surgical dentistry requires careful planning. Preoperative assessment and planning of all extractions needs to be thorough. Surgical extractions are best avoided and any tooth at risk of fracture or decoronation should be planned as a surgery-based procedure rather than a domiciliary one. All dental treatment runs the risk of producing emergencies and any interventive treatment can fail, so contingencies must be considered. If restorations are planned, consider the implications for post-operative pain or infection and any need for emergency recall. Avoid carrying out deep restorations on a Friday afternoon if there is a risk of post-operative pulpitis as it is unlikely that local weekend emergency dental services will cater for domiciliary visits. The adage "failing to plan is planning to fail" is most apt in the domiciliary situation.

Health and Safety

Dental staff can be vulnerable during domiciliary visits and personal safety issues must be considered. Protocols need to be devised to minimise risk. All visits must be prearranged. A pre-visit telephone call is useful to let the individual know that you will be arriving shortly. Carriage of a mobile telephone is recommended and a copy of the visiting schedule should be left back at base for reference. Visits should always be in pairs and identification should be shown before entering any premises. Some residences may be deemed too high a risk to visit. The entry bell panel for a block of flats where a domiciliary dental visit had been requested is shown in Fig 2-13. Only flat 7 was legally occupied with the other flats being derelict and local police had warned against entering the property following incidents in the unoccupied flats.

Domiciliary visits take place in a number of different environments, including, care homes, day centres, private residences, local hospitals and palliative care units. Each location presents a different set of health and safety hazards to the dental team. A risk assessment needs to be made to ensure a safe working environment that provides the patient with privacy.

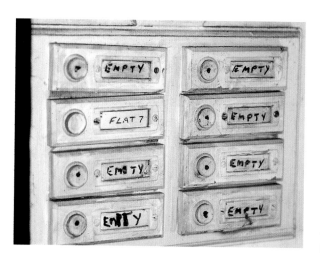

Fig 2-13 Bell panel of block of flats – only flat 7 occupied.

Infection Control

Maintaining good infection control can be a challenge in the domiciliary setting, but should follow the same principles as in the surgery, including:

- Zoning – clearly identify "clean" and "dirty" zones.
- Barrier coverings – use cling-film or plastic-backed disposable towels on any surfaces on which materials are mixed or placed.
- Transport instrument sets in metal instrument trays with lids.
- Procedural instrument trays are good practice: these are based on a "unit dose" concept where all the reusable instruments necessary for a procedure are kept in a single container and returned to it at the end of the treatment.
- Return sharp items to the surgery for disposal using the lidded instrument trays.
- Used equipment, laboratory items and clinical waste must be transported back to the surgery for disposal and decontamination in rigid, closed containers (Fig 2-11).
- Tape and seal tray systems for transport to avoid loose instruments emerging during travel.
- Implement a strict segregation policy of clean and contaminated material and equipment to ensure that clinical waste from one visit does not come into contact with equipment for a subsequent visit.

Medical Emergencies

The risks of medical emergencies occurring during domiciliary visits are no less likely than in a surgery setting. In fact the nature of the patient's age and/or medical condition puts them in a higher risk category for medical emergencies. There is just as much risk of a patient having an allergic reaction to latex in the home as in the dental surgery. In the domiciliary setting, it is prudent to use latex-free items, including gloves, routinely. Standard items of medical emergency equipment are required. Portable oxygen delivery systems along with emergency equipment such as airways, portable suction, a positive pressure ventilating device and a standard selection of emergency drugs are readily available for domiciliary use.

A portable "D"-sized oxygen cylinder with attachments for positive pressure, suction and airways is shown in Fig 2-14. It is necessary to have them on hand and quickly accessible and you must judge when to transport them from the car to the home (e.g. if your vehicle is parked directly outside the patient's home), they could be left in the boot of the car.

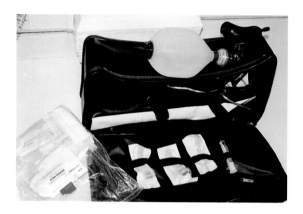

Fig 2-14 Portable oxygen, suction and airways.

Mobile Dental Units

Some salaried dental services have mobile units to which patients can be referred. This usually comprises a fully equipped dental vehicle that is essentially a walk-in dental surgery and delivers a service inside the van. The advantages of this service are that they provide easy access to a conventional dental setting and can supply all types of dental treatment. The main disadvantage is the cost of setting up the service. It is more likely to visit care homes or day centres than individuals at home, as this minimises difficulties with travelling, parking, setting up and accessing power sources whilst maximising the numbers of patients treated in a defined time period.

Conclusions

- Access to oral healthcare by people with physical disabilities requires a thorough assessment of your working environment, whether it is surgery or domiciliary based.
- Changes to the surgery environment and the provision of any domiciliary dentistry need to be carefully planned and organised.
- Always consider the impact of the individual's disability on their ability to maintain oral health; assess the impact of dental treatment upon their disability; and adopt a flexible approach that tailors treatment to the patient's individual needs.

Further Reading

Fiske J. Chronic Neurological Disease in Oral Medicine in Oral Care. In: Davies A (ed.). Advanced Disease. Oxford: Oxford University Press, 2005.

Fiske J, Hyland K. Parkinson's disease and oral care. Dent Update 2000; 27:58-65.

Fiske J, Lewis D. The development of standards for domiciliary dental care services: Guidelines and recommendations. Gerodontology 2000;17:119-122.

Fiske J, Griffiths J, Thompson S. Multiple sclerosis and oral care. Dent Update 2002;29:273-283.

French S. On equal terms: working with disabled people. Oxford: Butterworth-Heinemann, 1994.

Chapter 3
Managing the Patient With a Sensory Disability

Aim

The aim of this chapter is to increase awareness and understanding about the management of people with visual impairment, hearing impairment and the combination of both known as "deaf blindness".

Outcome

After reading this chapter you should have an understanding of the common causes of visual and auditory impairments, the demography of these conditions and the most appropriate ways of communicating with people affected by these conditions.

Introduction

Communication is a complex system of sending, receiving, and interpreting messages that relies, to a great extent, on seeing, hearing or both. If either or both of these sensory systems are impaired, the communication process can be damaged. This can have a profound effect on access to dental services by complicating the appointment-making process. In the dental setting the ability to glean essential information during history taking, to build patient rapport and trust, and the provision of effective preventive information can be impaired. The communication process can become time-consuming and frustrating for all involved if it is not well managed.

Visual and auditory impairments may be congenital, inherited, or acquired throughout life as the result of accident, disease, or as part of the ageing process.

Visual Impairments

Visual impairment refers to those people who have a visual disability that cannot be corrected by spectacles. It includes people who are entitled to register as blind or partially sighted, have difficulty reading an ordinary-print newspaper, or whose sight restricts their mobility. Most visually impaired people have some useful residual sight and only 4% cannot distinguish between light and dark.

Partial sightedness refers to people who cannot clearly see how many fingers are being held up at a distance of 6 metres or less (even with their glasses or lenses).

Blindness occurs when a person is unable to clearly see how many fingers are being held up at a distance of 3 metres or less (even with their glasses or lenses). However, they may still have some degree of vision (Table 3-1).

Table 3-1 **Classification of visual impairment using visual acuity**

Visual acuity	**Visual impairment**
VA 6/12 to > 6/18	Disruptive to lifestyle; may be unable to drive; difficulty reading small print and recognising a friend across the street, even when wearing glasses
VA 6/18 to better than 3/60	Severe sight problem. Partially sighted and can only read the top letter of the eye chart from six metres or less
VA < 3/60	Registered as blind and can only read the top letter of the eye chart from three metres or less

Demography: In the UK it is estimated that there are:
- About 1.7 million people over the age of 65 with sight problems. This represents 90% of all visually impaired people. Most of this group have lost their sight gradually, and many have an additional disability or illness.
- Approximately 25,000 children have sight problems and about 12,000 of these children also have other disabilities.
- 378,000 people are registered as blind or partially sighted.

Aetiology: The symptoms of sight loss depend greatly on the cause and can be due to disease, nerve damage or accidents. Common causes of visual impairment are:

- *Macular degeneration:* This accounts for about 50% of all registerable visual impairment and is the most common cause of poor sight in peo-

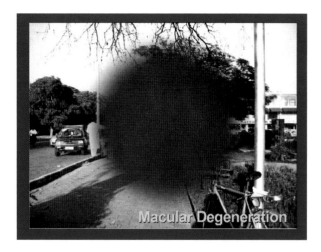

Fig 3-1 Macular degeneration.

ple over the age of 60. It usually involves both eyes, although they may not be affected at the same time. The macula, at the centre of the retina, which is used for detailed activities such as reading, recognising faces, and detecting colours is affected. In the early stages, central vision may be blurred or distorted, with objects looking an unusual size or shape and straight lines appearing wavy or fuzzy. This may happen quickly or develop over several months. There may be extreme sensitivity to light or the person may see lights, shapes and colours that are not there. As it becomes advanced, the individual will often notice a blank patch or dark spot in the centre of their sight. This makes reading, writing and recognising faces or small objects difficult. Age-related macular degeneration is not painful, and rarely leads to total blindness. People usually retain sufficient peripheral vision to be able to get around and maintain their independence (Fig 3-1).

- **Cataracts:** These can form at any age, but most often develop as people get older. In younger people cataracts can result from conditions such as diabetes, certain medications and other long-standing eye problems. A cataract is one or more opacity of the crystalline lens. The opacification of the lens may occur in different ways, so that the light rays which reach the retina may be split, causing multiple images. Having cataracts has been likened to looking through a dirty windscreen – if the sun is behind you, your view is reasonably good, but if the sun is in front of you, then your view can be seriously impaired (Fig 3-2). Approximately 50% of people between 65 and 74 years of age and 70% of people over the age of 75 have cataracts.

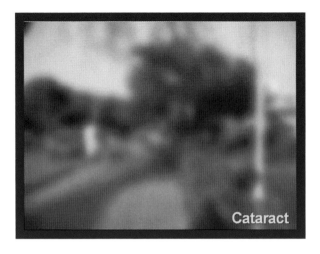

Fig 3-2 Cataract.

They can experience:
- decreased visual acuity
- decreased contrast sensitivity leading to difficulty seeing in poorly lit environments
- increased sensitivity to light and glare
- blurred distance vision
- difficulty reading
- difficulty with colour contrast
- double vision.

Cataract surgery has a high success rate and 95% of patients experience improved vision if there are no other eye conditions present.

- *Diabetic retinopathy*: This is the largest single cause of registerable visual impairment among people of working age. The probability of a visual impairment is greatly increased if the diabetes is poorly controlled. In diabetic retinopathy the fine network of fragile blood vessels in the retina may leak or become blocked, causing local loss of function. At first, there will be a few specks of blood, or spots, "floating" in the field of vision (Fig 3-3). Bleeding can reoccur and cause severely blurred vision. It can cause double vision and difficulty focusing. If left untreated, proliferative retinopathy can cause severe vision loss and even blindness. Other side-effects of diabetes include poor circulation and peripheral neuropathy; these can result in poor tactual sensitivity which means that people with diabetes may not be able to read Braille.

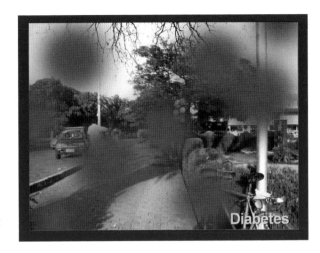

Fig 3-3 Diabetic retinopathy.

- *Glaucoma:* There are several types of glaucoma. Congenital glaucoma appears in young people, primary glaucoma is most frequently associated with ageing, and secondary glaucoma is the result of injury or trauma. It is uncommon below the age of 40 but affects 1% of people over the age of 40 years and 5% of people over the age of 65. People over the age of 60, of African origin and over the age of 40, and people with a family history of glaucoma are at risk of developing glaucoma. It impairs vision by creating pressure that damages the optic nerve. The first problems are with peripheral vision. As it progresses, it can destroy all peripheral vision causing tunnel vision, and eventually impairing central vision leading to total blindness (Fig 3-4).

Treatments for glaucoma are aimed at bringing down the pressure in the eye to a level that is low enough to prevent harm to the optic nerve. Once the optic nerve is damaged, lowering the pressure only prevents further damage. With tunnel vision, it is often possible to read small print, but not large print.

Recognition: People with a visual impairment may be recognisable because they have difficulty reading, wear specialised glasses, carry a white cane or stick, and/or are accompanied by a guide dog (Fig 3-5).

If you recognise a person as visually impaired, ask how much residual vision they have and what their preferred method of communication is and record this information in the notes.

31

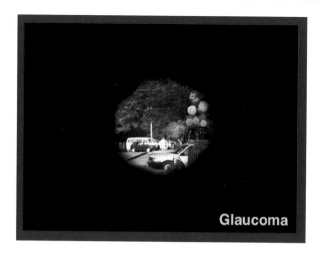

Fig 3-4 Glaucoma – tunnel vision.

Support: Tactile feedback, such as a handshake on meeting, can make people with a visual impairment feel more comfortable. Guide the person through the practice by allowing them to take hold of your elbow rather than taking them by the arm. Warn them if you are coming to any steps

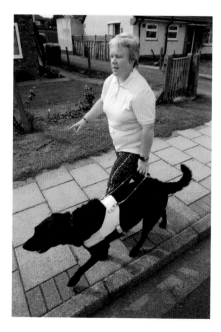

Fig 3-5 Woman with guide dog.

and say how many. If they have a guide or assistance dog, check whether their dog will remain in the waiting room or accompany them into the surgery. Dogs of this nature are well trained and behaved and are not startled by loud or sudden noises such as the air-rotor or high-volume aspirator.

Communication: To communicate effectively with visually impaired people you need to consider printed material (including letters, appointment cards and information sheets), signage in the practice, and alternative ways of presenting information such as spoken word, cassette or CD, and tactile formats such as Braille.

Written material: Guidance such as the Royal National Institute for the Blind "Clear Print" guidelines recommend: the use of matt paper, a plain background, a strongly contrasting print colour, font size 14 or more, a weight of type sufficient for easy reading, such as Arial, and text in mixed case rather than capitals.

Signage: This should be prominent, at eye level and follow the same rules as for printed materials. Light text or illustrations can be used on a dark background provided there is good contrast, and non-reflective materials should always be used.

Speaking: When speaking to the individual, face them and ensure that there is no strong back lighting as this interferes with residual vision. Keep them informed of each step in the procedure, especially when there is about to be a sudden noise or sensation. Try to describe procedures in terms of how they will sound and feel.

Auditory Impairments

"Deaf" is a general term used to refer to people with all degrees of hearing loss. The level of deafness is defined according to the quietest sound a person can hear, measured in decibels:

- Mild deafness: the quietest sounds that can be heard are 25–39 decibels. It can cause difficulty following speech in noisy situations.
- Moderate deafness: the quietest sounds that can be heard are 40–69 decibels. It can cause difficulty following speech without a hearing aid.
- Severe deafness: the quietest sounds that can be heard are 70–94 decibels. People may rely on lip-reading even with a hearing aid. British sign language may be the preferred method of communication.
- Profound deafness: the quietest sounds that can be heard are 95 decibels or more. British sign language may be the preferred method of communication.

Demography: In the majority of developed countries, most deaf and hard of hearing people (approximately 1 in 7 of the population) have developed a hearing loss as they aged. A relatively small number of children are born with significant deafness every year. Only about 2% of young adults are deaf or hard of hearing. Around the age of 50 the proportion of deaf people begins to increase sharply and 55% of people over 60 are deaf or hard of hearing. By way of example, data for the UK are shown in Table 3-2. Approximately 698,000 people are severely or profoundly deaf. Another 450,000 cannot hear well enough to use a voice telephone, even with equipment to make it louder. However, people who cannot use voice telephones can use text-phones or videophones.

Aetiology: Deafness has many causes:
- Congenital deafness occurs in around 1 in every 16,000 births. Autosomal recessive inheritance accounts for more than 75% of cases, although only around 20% of cases are associated with syndromes. Complications during pregnancy such as infection from measles, rubella, or cytomegaloviruses and a range of ototoxic drugs can damage hearing before birth. Post-natal causes in infancy include premature birth, childhood infections (e.g. meningitis, measles and mumps) and ototoxic drugs, used to treat other types of infections in babies.
- Head injury.
- Exposure to loud noise.
- Age-associated deafness – 50% of people over the age of 60 having some degree of hearing loss.
- Tinnitus, a sensation of ringing in the ears, is often associated with deafness.

Table 3-2 **Estimated percentages of the UK population who are deaf or hard of hearing**

Age	16 to 60 years	61 to 80 years	> 80 years
Mild deafness	4.6%	28.1%	18.4%
Moderate deafness	1.6%	16.5%	57.9%
Severe deafness	0.2%	1.9%	13.2%
Profound deafness	0.1%	0.4%	3.6%
All degrees of deafness	6.5%	46.9%	93.1%

Types of deafness: There are two types of deafness:
- *Conductive deafness* or otitis media is most common. It is caused by fluid building up in the middle ear preventing sound from passing efficiently through the middle ear to the cochlea and auditory nerve. Most conductive deafness is temporary but it can become permanent.
- *Sensori-neural deafness* is caused by a fault in the inner ear or auditory nerve. It is usually caused by a problem in the cochlea and is permanent.

Tinnitus: It is estimated that 1 in 5 people experiences some degree of "ringing" ears or other head noises perceived in the absence of any external noise source. These noises may be continuous or intermittent; vary in pitch from a low roar to a high squeal or whine; and occur unilaterally or bilaterally. When the ringing or noise is constant it is annoying, distracting, and can cause trouble with hearing despite there being no associated deafness. Tinnitus and deafness can coexist.

Recognition: Unless a patient is wearing a hearing aid or informs you that they do not hear well, there may be no signs to indicate deafness. Because deafness is perceived as being equated with stupidity by society, deaf people may attempt to hide their disability. They can be quite skilled at answering yes/no questions. It may only be when you ask for more detail that you realise the person does not hear well.

Support: If you recognise a person as deaf, ask them what their preferred method of communication is and record it in the notes.

Communication: When communicating with a hearing-impaired person improve your chances of success and reduce the chances of frustration by:
- positioning yourself with your face to the light so you can be clearly seen
- facing the patient so they can read your lips
- removing your facemask or wearing a clear face shield to facilitate reading of lips and facial expression
- eliminating background noise, such as music
- minimising interruptions
- giving the patient extra time to respond
- changing the phraseology you use if it is not understood rather than repeating the same words
- speaking clearly in a slightly louder voice than normal if necessary
- resisting the urge to shout – it won't help
- lowering the pitch of your voice – this can be more effective than raising your voice as people lose high-pitch hearing first

- using visual feedback through gestures (e.g. nodding or shaking your head for yes or no, or a thumbs up for you are doing well)
- being prepared to write down what you have to say
- having pre-prepared written prompts to save time.

If the patient relies on:

- *Hearing aids:* Ensure that their hearing aid is switched on. People often turn hearing aids off before coming into the dental surgery, in anticipation of the high-pitched whistling interference that may occur when in close proximity to the dentist and some dental equipment. You may need to ask them to switch the aid back on for periods of communication.
- *Lip-reading:* By following the general communication guidance and speaking clearly in a normal cadence and tone, it is usually possible for people to lip-read.
- *British Sign Language (BSL):* This tends to be used by people who were born deaf. BSL (recognised as a language in its own right in March 2003) uses manual and non-manual components, such as hand shapes and movements, facial expression, and shoulder movement. Unless someone in the practice can sign, you will need an interpreter to attend the appointment. Ideally, meet the interpreter in advance of the appointment to discuss dental terminology and interpretation needs (Fig 3-6).

There are other technical aids that can help to overcome hearing impairments and improve access to dental care, for example minicom text machines and induction hearing loops.

Deafblindness

Deafblind people have a combined sight and hearing loss, which leads to difficulties in communicating, mobility, and accessing information. Deafblindness has been described as one of the loneliest conditions in the world. Understanding your surroundings without sight or hearing, and the general lack of understanding of the disability, can lead to feelings of isolation and helplessness.

Demography: Deafblindness is not common, for example there are in the order of 24,000 deafblind people in the UK. This is approximately 0.05% of the population. Some of these people will be totally deaf and totally blind, others will have some residual hearing and/or vision. However, these figures do not take into account the large number of older people who are losing

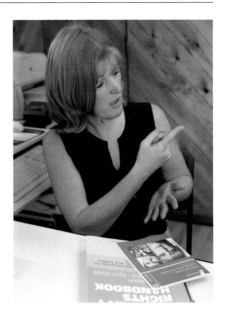

Fig 3-6 Woman using sign language.

both their sight and hearing. Consequently, the number of people with a combined sight and hearing loss multiplies tenfold.

Aetiology: Deafblindness can be congenital or acquired.

Congenital – The main causes are:
- Rubella (German measles) contracted during the first trimester of pregnancy. The advent of vaccination has led to a decrease in deafblindness from Rubella infection.
- Premature birth and difficulties in labour are now more common causes of deafblindness. They may be linked to infections during pregnancy or rare genetic disorders.

It is common for people with congenital deafblindness to have other disabilities, such as learning difficulties, epilepsy, and severe physical disabilities.

Acquired – The main causes are:
- Usher syndrome – a genetic condition that causes congenital deafness or hearing and sight loss over a number of years usually commences in late childhood. The sight loss is due to retinitis pigmentosa and results in tunnel vision. It affects 3–6% of people born deaf or partially hearing. They often do not realise they have Usher syndrome until they begin to lose their sight. Coming to terms with the additional loss of vision can be extremely difficult and

may lead to emotional and psychological difficulties. The syndrome is not associated with learning difficulties or other physical disabilities.
- Accident and illness affecting people who were born deaf or blind causing them to lose their sight or hearing.
- Ageing accounts for the largest group of people who develop deafblindness. Around 50% of people over 75 years of age who have a visual impairment will also have a hearing deficit. This dual sensory loss can lead to depression, and difficulties with daily living activities.

Recognition: People who are blind and deaf may carry a white and red cane so that their disability can be recognised. Unfortunately most people are unaware of its meaning.

Support: The support that an individual requires will depend on when they developed their dual sensory loss.
- People born deafblind (with or without additional disabilities) require specialist services to meet their needs. They can find it difficult to communicate, to understand the concept of language, and are likely to be taught to communicate through the use of symbols, objects of reference, sign language, Braille, etc.
- People who have adapted to visual impairment during their lives and are now losing their hearing may need to rely on tactile sign language.
- Older people with hearing loss, whose usual means of communication relies on lip-reading or sign language who are now losing their sight may require large print initially and reach a stage where they too rely on a tactile form of sign language.

Communication: It is always advisable to ask the individual, or their carer, what is their preferred method of communication. This may involve sign language, telecommunications equipment, or the use of an interpreter. Deafblind people who were born deaf or went deaf in early years usually use British Sign Language, rather than spoken English. A significant proportion of deafblind people still have a little useful sight and hearing which can be assisted by wearing glasses and hearing aids. However, if there is a lot of background noise, hearing aids magnify this, making it difficult to pick out the speaker's voice. Also, if the person relies on lip-reading, good lighting is essential, or they cannot "see" what the speaker is saying.

Deafblind UK provides an information sheet that provides two simple methods of sign language in visual form for easy learning and/or reference. Both systems require words to be spelled out:

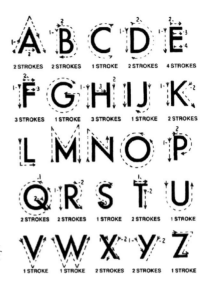

Fig 3-7 The Block Alphabet. The dotted lines indicate the direction and sequence of strokes to be made on the palm.

- The "Block Alphabet" is a system whereby you use a forefinger to trace ordinary block capital letters on the palm of the deafblind person's hand. Each letter is traced directly on top of the last. The information sheet shows the direction and sequence of strokes required for each letter (Fig 3-7).
- The "Deafblind Manual Alphabet" is a quicker method and is like the finger spelling used in British Sign Language, but placed on the hand. Different letters are spelt out by touching specific areas of the fingertips and palm of the deafblind person.

Quick signs for Yes and No are as follows:
- Yes – a double "y" is 2 taps on the deafblind person's palm of the hand with your first finger, and
- No – your first two fingers onto the deafblind person's palm (as for n) and rub left to right twice.

The deafblind manual can be learnt in half an hour and after practice it can be possible to have a conversation at a reasonable pace by using this type of finger spelling (Fig 3-8). Deafblind people with a little sight need large print to be able to read it. Others who are blind need their information in a tactile form such as Braille (Fig 3-9) or Moon (Fig 3-10) which they can read with their fingertips. Those who have residual hearing may prefer to have information provided on audio cassette.

Assistance: You can assist a deafblind person by:
- finding out their preferred mode of communication and using it
- remembering that the person is deaf and blind – not stupid
- guiding the person through the practice by letting them hold your arm
- approaching them gently and tapping their arm to let them know you are there
- not walking off suddenly and leaving the person stranded.

A touch the top of the person's thumb

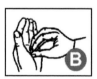

B - make an o-shape with all your fingers and thumb. Place the tips into the palm of the deaf-blind person

N - lay your first two fingers across the person's palm, ensuring that your fingers are held together. If the fingers are not held together, it may feel like a V

Fig 3-8 Letters from the Deafblind Alphabet Manual.

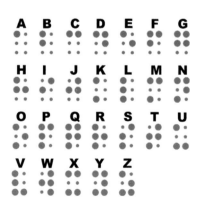

Fig 3-9 The Braille Alphabet.

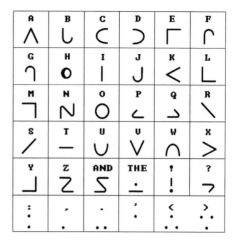

Fig 3-10 The Moon Alphabet.

Conclusions

- Sensory disabilities are common and you need to be prepared to deal with people who have them.
- Design changes to your practice with people with sensory disability in mind. That way everyone's needs are met.
- When you have a patient with sensory disability, ensure that you ascertain, record, and use the individual's preferred mode of communication.

Useful Contacts:

Royal National Institute for the Deaf (RNID) www.rnid.org.uk
Royal National Institute for the Blind (RNIB) www.rnib.org.uk
Sense (UK deafblind charity) www.sense.org.uk

Deafblind UK www.deafblind.org.uk

Council for the Advancement of Communication with Deaf People (CACDP) www.cacdp.org.uk

Sign Solutions www.signsolutions.uk.com

British Sign Language www.britishsignlanguage.com

Chapter 4

Managing the Patient With a Learning Disability

Aim

The aim of this chapter is to outline the common causes of learning disability and how they impact on oral health and patient management.

Outcome

After reading this chapter you will have an understanding of the common conditions associated with learning disability, and how it impacts on oral health and its management. You will also understand the issues related to consent and patient management.

Introduction

Learning disability is a significant impairment of intelligence and social functioning acquired before adulthood. Its cause can be genetic, congenital, or acquired.

Learning disability affects the way someone learns, communicates and carries out everyday activities. The amount of support a person requires throughout life varies according to the severity of their learning disability and whether or not they have additional physical disability. People with a mild learning disability may need little support, whereas those with severe learning disability may need support with all types of daily living activities. However, people with a learning disability can learn and achieve with the right support.

Demography

In most developed countries around 2.5% of the population have a learning disability. In the UK this equates to 1.5 to 2 million people. Of these people, 200,000 (10%) have a severe or profound disability. Almost 15% of this subgroup (over 29,000 people with a severe or profound learning disability) live at home with carers aged over 70 years of age. Overall, more males are affected by learning disability than females.

Additional Disabilities

People with learning disabilities have an increased prevalence of associated disabilities including:
- physical impairments
- sensory impairments
- behavioural problems
- epilepsy
- congenital heart defects, and
- mental health problems.

25% of people with a learning disability are profoundly disabled with additional disabilities.

Causes

The commonest causes of learning disability are Down's syndrome and Fragile X syndrome. It also occurs in Velo-Cardio-Facial (or DiGeorge) syndrome. Learning disability is commonly associated with the spectrum of autistic disorders.

1. Down's Syndrome (DS) is a genetic condition caused by a chromosomal abnormality (usually trisomy of chromosome 21) that results in a characteristic appearance and learning disability, which ranges from mild to severe. There are currently more than 26,000 people in the UK with DS where its incidence is 1.5 per 1000 births. Its prevalence is likely to rise in the coming decades because life expectancy of people with DS has improved dramatically.

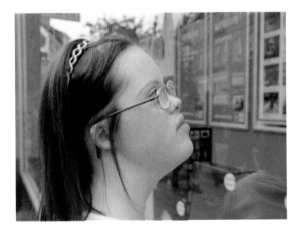

Fig 4-1 Characteristic appearance in Down's syndrome.

Characteristic appearance – of short stature, relatively short arms and legs, broad hands and short fingers, flattened face and occiput, slanting eyes and prominent epicanthic folds, and underdevelopment of the middle third of face and relative prognathism (Fig 4-1).

Oro-dental characteristics – include delayed development and eruption of both dentitions, hypodontia, microdontia, hypocalcification and hypoplastic defects, occlusal problems, and a high incidence of severe early onset periodontal disease. Mouth breathing, which may occur because of smaller nasal passages, contributes to increased gingival inflammation around anterior teeth.

General features – include cardiac anomalies (40%), vision impairments (50%), hearing impairment (mild to moderate in 50%), atlanto-axial instability or subluxation (20%), compromised immune system, hypothyroidism, increased risk of epilepsy, and increased risk of Alzheimer's disease (45% of people reaching the age of 55).

Considerations for oral health and dental treatment – required as a result of general health features are outlined in Table 4-1.

2. Fragile X Syndrome (FXS) is the most common cause of *inherited* learning disability occurring in approximately 1 in 3600 males and 1 in 4000 to 6000 females. It is also the most common known cause of autism, being responsible for 2–6% of all cases. Approximately one third of all children diagnosed with FXS have autism. FXS symptoms also can include characteristic physical and behavioural features and delays in speech and language development.

Males are more severely affected than females. The majority of males with FXS have a significant intellectual disability and a variety of physical and behavioural characteristics. Physical features such as enlarged ears and a long face with a prominent chin are common. Connective tissue problems may include ear infections, mitral valve prolapse, flat feet, double-jointed fingers, hyperflexible joints and a variety of skeletal problems. Behavioural characteristics in males include attention deficit disorders, speech disturbances, hand biting, hand flapping, autistic behaviours, poor eye contact, and unusual responses to various touch, auditory or visual stimuli. Females usually have milder intellectual disability and presentation of the behavioural or physical features. About a third of the females have a significant intellectual disability. Similarly, the physical and behavioural characteristics are often expressed to a lesser degree.

3. Velo-Cardio-Facial Syndrome (VCFS) or DiGeorge syndrome is due to a missing piece of genetic information on the long arm of one of chromosomes 22. It is estimated that around 1 in 3000–4000 births are affected. As

Table 4-1 **Impact of general health on oral health/dental treatment in Down's syndrome** (continued over page)

General condition	Implications for oral health/dental treatment
Cardiac anomalies (congenital in children, and mitral valve prolapse in adults)	• If not corrected with surgery during infancy, need for antibiotic prophylaxis for invasive dental treatment • Plan treatment to minimise the number of antibiotic episodes required • Instigation of a preventive strategy to reduce the risk of developing dental disease and the need for invasive treatment
Visual impairment (including myopia, hyperopia, astigmatism and cataracts)	• Can affect the person's ability to carry out effective oral hygiene • May need to enlist the help of a carer
Hearing impairment (as a result of middle ear infections and fluid accumulation)	• May not hear instructions • May need to use an alternative form of communication
Atlanto-axial joint instability	• Do not hyperextend the neck as this can cause irreversible damage to the spinal cord • It may influence the individual's cooperation of reclining in the dental chair • Investigate status prior to a general anaesthetic
Compromised immune system	• Predisposition to periodontal disease, aphthous ulcers and candidiasis • Instigate preventive strategy • Increased susceptibility to infections, particularly of the skin, gastrointestinal and respiratory systems • Need to treat infections aggressively

Table 4-1 **Impact of general health on oral health/dental treatment in Down's syndrome** (continued)

General condition	Implications for oral health/dental treatment
Epilepsy	• Possible side-effects of medication (e.g. dry mouth, gingival hyperplasia if taking phenytoin, increased caries if syrup-based) • Ensure seizure and drug histories are current
Alzheimer's disease	• Short-term memory loss • Progressive loss of daily living skills • Decreased ability to cope and cooperate with dental treatment and oral hygiene • May need to enlist the help of a carer

its name suggests the common features are cleft palate, congenital heart defect (CHD), and characteristic facial appearance (elongated face, almond-shaped eyes, wide nose, and small ears). It is the most common cause of CHD after Down's syndrome. Learning disability and communication difficulties similar to those associated with autism also occur.

4. Autistic Spectrum Disorders (ASD) affect 1 in 1000 of the population and occur more frequently in males than in females (3.5:1). It is a lifelong developmental disability that affects the way a person communicates and relates to people around them. About 70% of people with ASD have the same intellectual function as people without ASD, but they all share a difficulty in making sense of the world. They have a triad of impairments affecting social interaction, social communication and imagination (Table 4-2). People with ASD sometimes have additional disabilities, such as epilepsy, sensory impairments, Down's syndrome, and physical disabilities.

Epilepsy and Learning Disability

Epilepsy, which occurs in less than 1% of the general population, affects in the order of 30% of people with a learning disability. The more severe the learning disability, the more likely the person is to have epilepsy. At least 50% of people with severe learning disability also have epilepsy. It occurs in around 2%

Table 4-2 **The triad of impairments**

Social interaction – difficulty with social relationships	Social communication – difficulty with verbal and non-verbal communication	Imagination
Appears aloof and indifferent to other people	Not fully understanding the meaning of gestures, facial expressions or tone of voice	Children have difficulty playing imaginatively with objects or other children/adults
A general preference for isolation in the presence of others	Failure to develop useful speech and its use	Activities might be copied and pursued rigidly and repetitively
Failure to seek comfort at times of distress	Difficulty in talking about feelings or thoughts	Shift from physical activities to the collection of information
Inability to understand social rules and conventions	Difficulty understanding the emotions, ideas and beliefs of others	Focus on minor or trivial aspects of things in the environment. Activity seems complex, but careful observation shows it is rigid and stereotyped in nature

of children with DS, increasing to 10% in adulthood. Seizure management and treatment are the same as for people without learning disability.

Oral Health

Learning disability can affect oral health through a person's ability to cope and cooperate with dental care, and through the inability to manage daily oral hygiene. Generally rates of caries and periodontal disease in people with a learning disability are comparable to the general population. Periodontal disease in DS, where an impaired immune system causes predisposition, is an exception to this general rule. However, the following factors may lead to increased caries, poorer periodontal conditions, and additional oral health problems in people with learning disability:

- long-term medications – sugar-based and/or with xerostomic side-effects
- unusual/faddy eating habits
- damaging oral habits such as bruxism, tongue thrusting, self-injurious behaviour
- poor manual dexterity, hindering effective oral hygiene
- inability to comply with carer for oral hygiene.

There is evidence that people with learning disability experience poorer oral health and worse oral healthcare outcomes than the general population, with less restored caries, more extractions, poorer oral hygiene and more severe periodontal disease.

It is important to work with parents/carers to ensure that a rigorous preventive regime is employed at home. They will need information, advice and support to maintain their motivation. You can help by:

- talking to them about brushing techniques and demonstrating them
- making advice pragmatic and appropriate, for example advising the use of chlorhexidine gels and high fluoride content pastes rather than mouth rinses for someone who cannot rinse and spit
- raising awareness about medicines with a high sugar content or xerostomic side-effects and giving practical advice
- discussing diet and how/if it might be changed to benefit oral health.

Consent

Obtaining informed consent for dental treatment is an ethical and legal responsibility. In order to do so, information, choice and capacity and competence need to be considered. In order to have the capacity to make competent decisions regarding their own care, an adult patient must be able to:

- comprehend information
- retain information pertinent to the decision
- understand the likely consequences of the decision.

Consent to treatment may be given by a parent or guardian for children under the age of 16 years. However, for people living in England and Wales aged 16 and over, no person may legally give consent to treatment on their behalf. In the case of people with learning disability, some will understand their dental treatment needs and be able to provide their own informed consent. Their ability to give informed consent may depend on the complexity of the treat-

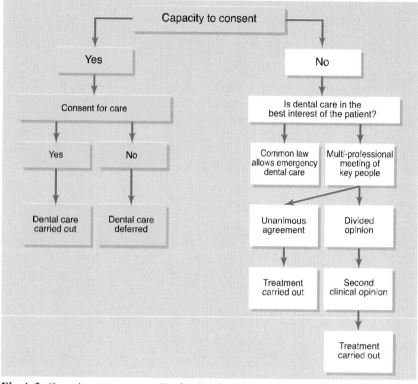

Fig 4-2 Capacity to consent – England and Wales.
Source: BSDH Guidelines. Principles on Intervention for People Unable to Comply with Routine Dental Care. 2004; www.bsdh.org.uk

ment and treatment implications. For example someone may understand that having an aching tooth removed will rid them of pain, yet not understand the implications for replacement of the tooth. Where a person's capacity to consent is compromised, it is good practice to obtain agreement to treatment from parents or carers. A "best interests" meeting may need to be called in order to do this. The law considers this good practice even though it has no legal status. However, it is also prudent to gain "professional agreement" (the consensus view of two dental practitioners) that the proposed treatment is in the best interests of the individual (Fig 4-2).

It is important to be aware of national legislation on consent. For example, in line with the Adults with Incapacity Act (Scotland) 2000, in Scotland a patient who is not capable of informed consent must have a completed Certificate of Incapacity prior to provision of treatment. The proposed Mental Capacity Act 2007 may change current practice in England.

Patient Management

Achieving patient cooperation is based on building trust and rapport through the use of behavioural management techniques such as acclimatisation and "tell–show–do". The degree to which this is successful in people with a learning disability may depend on the severity of the learning disability. The following facts need to be taken into account and acted on accordingly:

- Compliance may not be static and may vary with different procedures and on different days.
- Acclimatisation, behaviour modification and constancy may improve compliance for some people but not all.
- There will be known triggers for behaviour change in some individuals and these should be avoided.
- The timing of appointments, medication and other aspects of daily routine, may be crucial.
- The use of less conventional relaxation techniques, for example, music therapy, may be beneficial.

The following set of principles can be useful in the management of patients with a learning disability:

- Talk with the parent or carer to determine your patient's intellectual and functional abilities.
- Plan one or more preliminary appointments to help the patient become familiar with the practice, the staff, and equipment.
- Communicate with the patient at a level they can understand.
- Always include the patient in any communication.
- Smile and use reassuring gestures and touch as appropriate.
- Make appointments short and positive.
- Begin a cursory oral examination using a toothbrush, as this is a familiar object to most patients and signals what comes next.
- Use a toothbrush to brush the teeth and to gain additional access to the patient's mouth.
- Keep dental instruments out of sight until needed.
- Use a "tell–show–do" approach:
  – explain each procedure before it occurs
  – show what you have explained
  – carry out the treatment.

- Always be honest but use non-emotive words.
- Keep the operating light out of your patient's eyes.
- Praise and reinforce good behaviour.
- Ignore inappropriate behaviour if possible.
- Maintain a consistent approach and setting.
- Resort to sedation or general anaesthesia only after trying behaviour management.

Communication

It is important to find out the best way of communicating with your patient. Some people with learning disability communicate using sign language such as Makaton (which has both hand signs and printed symbols). There is a helpful Makaton book called *Going to the Dentist* which can be used to help communication and to prepare patients for what will happen at future dental visits (see Further Reading).

Routines are very important to people with VCFS and ASD, and it can be important to say the same things in the same way. Their lack of social-interaction skills and the absence of abstract reasoning hampers communication. People with these syndromes think literally, so statements such as "you're driving me up the wall" are confusing and nonsensical and may even be interpreted as lying. They can also have difficulty remembering multi-step directions and can have disorganised thinking so that they become obsessed with one topic or idea. Making choices is difficult, so it is best to only ask one thing at a time; for example, instead of asking "Would you prefer a red toothbrush or a blue one?" just say "Would you like a red toothbrush?". Visual information can be easier to cope with than the spoken word and using photos, line drawings and symbols, simple written instructions or even text messages can be helpful.

Restraint and Physical Intervention

On occasions, where other behaviour management strategies have failed, some form of intervention will be required. Physical intervention; oral, intravenous and inhalation sedation; or general anaesthesia used as adjuncts to facilitate dental care are all a form of clinical restraint. There are times when reasonable physical intervention (restraint) is preferable to more extreme alternatives and might be acceptable for single, short interventions. Such an approach should only be countenanced when all other approaches have been exhausted.

If it is anticipated that physical intervention may be required, the patient should be assessed beforehand for any contraindications to its use. For example, patients with a history of heart disease, difficulty in breathing, a history of recent fractures or dislocated joints, and people with DS who have atlanto-axial joint instability. Once it is decided that a physical intervention is to be used in order to effectively accomplish the task, it must be:

- the minimum to be effective
- considered beneficial to the individual in completing the treatment
- neither seen nor used as a punishment nor convenience
- unlikely to cause physical trauma
- unlikely to cause more than minimum psychological trauma
- a means to avoid more severe forms of restraint, for example, general anaesthesia
- to avoid injury to the patient and/or others (e.g. to control involuntary movements)
- agreed, wherever possible, with those close to the patient, remembering that the clinician is ultimately responsible through the duty of care.

The following should be noted in the patient's record:
- the oral/dental procedure carried out
- the type of physical intervention
- the people consulted about the decision to use physical intervention
- the outcome and future plans.

In circumstances where the patient becomes distressed, treatment should be discontinued and plans discussed with the parent/carer about further attempts on a different day, or the use of a different form of clinical restraint such as sedation or general anaesthesia.

Conclusions

- Learning disability is common and can be compounded by other disabilities, such as epilepsy, that will also require appropriate management.
- Learning disability can impact adversely on oral health without support and management from an empathic dental team.
- The proper procedure for informed consent must be followed prior to commencing dental treatment.

Further Reading

BSDH Guidelines 2004. Principles on Intervention for People Unable to Comply with Routine Dental Care. www.bsdh.org.uk

Henwood S, Wilson MA, Edwards I. The role of competence and capacity in relation to consent for treatment in adult patients. Br Dent J 2006;200(1):18-21.

Steele, P et al. Going to the Dentist. Ballymena: Homefirst Community Trust, 2001.

Chapter 5
Managing the Patient With Mental Illness

Aim

The aim of this chapter is to increase awareness and understanding of mental illness through three common conditions – schizophrenia, depression and dementia.

Outcome

After reading this chapter you should have an understanding of three common causes of mental illness – schizophrenia, depression and dementia – their signs and symptoms, their effects on oral health, and how to manage the oral care of people with these conditions. This will also give you a basic understanding of the management of any patient who develops mental illness.

Introduction

Mental illness is defined as a disorder of the brain that results in a disruption in a person's thinking, feeling/mood, ability to relate to others and the ability to work. Mental illness is common. It has been estimated that around 20% of adults will suffer from a clinically diagnosable mental illness in a given year, but less than half of them will suffer symptoms severe enough to disrupt their daily functioning. Mental illness can have a huge impact on the ability to carry out daily living activities, including accessing and coping with dental services and maintaining daily oral hygiene. Consequently, mental illness can impact on oral health. Oral conditions may also be presenting features of mental illness, particularly of depression. They include atypical facial pain, atypical odontalgia, burning mouth syndrome and disordered taste and salivation. Organic causes should always be considered first in any differential diagnosis.

1. Schizophrenia

Schizophrenia ranks amongst the top 10 causes of disability. It is a form of mental illness in which mental function is impaired to the degree that it interferes with the ability to meet the demands of everyday life and to maintain contact with reality. Insight is diminished or lost completely. Some people only have one episode of schizophrenia during a lifetime. Others have many episodes, but lead relatively normal lives during the interim periods. The individual with a recurring or continuous pattern of illness often does not fully recover normal functioning and requires long-term medication to manage the symptoms.

Cause
There is no known single cause. It is likely that the disorder is associated with an imbalance of the complex chemical systems of the brain. There is an underlying genetic vulnerability to developing it. For example, the child of a parent with schizophrenia has a 1 in 10 chance of developing it compared with the general population risk of 1 in 100. Even so, certain environmental factors are needed before the disorder manifests. These factors include family relationships, life events (both good and bad) and infection.

Signs and Symptoms
The world of people with schizophrenia is one of:
• Disordered perceptions of reality.
• Hallucinations and illusions – hallucinations may be auditory, visual, tactile, gustatory or olfactory. Hearing voices that other people do not hear is commonest. The voices may describe the person's activities, carry on a conversation, warn of impending dangers or issue orders.
• Delusions – these may be of persecution, false or irrational beliefs (e.g. of being cheated, harassed, poisoned or conspired against), or delusions of grandeur. They can be bizarre (e.g. believing that someone is controlling their behaviour with magnetic waves, or that their thoughts are being broadcast aloud).
• Disordered thinking – resulting in the inability to concentrate, being easily distracted, unable to focus attention, and unable to sort out what is and is not relevant to a situation. It can result in thought disorder.
• Blunted or flat emotional expression – such that a person may speak in a monotone voice, have diminished facial expression, and appear apathetic and withdrawn.

Management
The mainstay of treatment is the use of antipsychotic medication. Most people show dramatic improvement with these drugs. Their side-effects include:
• drowsiness or restlessness

- muscle spasms
- xerostomia – leading to increased risk of caries, periodontal disease, denture problems and oral infection
- tardive dyskinesia – a disorder characterised by involuntary movements most often affecting the jaws, lips and tongue causing involuntary movement of the tongue and facial grimacing that can lead to difficulties in the delivery of dental treatment and in wearing dentures
- agranulocytosis – the white blood count should be regularly monitored. Repeated dental infections could indicate a low white blood cell count.

Psychosocial treatments such as rehabilitation, individual psychotherapy, and family education and self-help groups are also used in the management of schizophrenia.

Nicotine
The most common form of substance misuse in people with schizophrenia (approximately 75–90%) is nicotine dependence through smoking. Whilst people smoke to self-mediate their symptoms, nicotine interferes with the response to antipsychotic drugs. Several studies have found that people with schizophrenia who smoke need higher doses of antipsychotic drugs. Heavy smoking has a detrimental effect on oral health.

Violence
Despite the common stereotype linking schizophrenia and violence, studies indicate that most people with schizophrenia are not prone to violence. The specific subgroups include:
- people with a record of criminal violence before becoming ill
- people with substance misuse or alcohol problems
- people with paranoid and psychotic symptoms.

Oral Health
People with schizophrenia have greater risk of oral diseases and have greater oral treatment needs. Generally there is a higher incidence of caries and worse periodontal conditions than in the general population. This is the result of a complex interrelationship of socioeconomic factors, illness, its treatment, deterioration in ability to self-care, habits such as poor diet and smoking, dental attendance, and barriers to access to oral care.

Dental Management
It is unlikely that an individual in an acute episode of their illness will seek dental care, and the majority of people with schizophrenia can be safely

treated in mainstream dental practice. People with chronically poorly controlled, or uncontrolled, schizophrenia require referral to a specialist dental service.

Challenges that this group of people may present to the dental team include:

- **Communication** – this can be difficult because of associated disordered thinking or because of auditory hallucinations. In the latter case, it is prudent to check if the patient has heard what you said. If their voices are talking to them, you will not have been heard.
- **Cooperation** – this may vary from patient to patient or from visit to visit for the same person. Gentle persuasion is worth trying but the individual's wishes need to be respected. If a patient is openly uncooperative or shows signs of aggression it is best to curtail the appointment as politely as possible.
- **Compliance** – little interest and/or ability to maintain oral hygiene is part of the condition when it is poorly controlled or uncontrolled. This can be frustrating to the dental team but it needs to be remembered that this is a feature of the illness.
- **Delusions** – it is recognised that some people with schizophrenia have believed that they receive radio transmissions from amalgam fillings. If a non-metallic restorative material can be used, this is a safer option. Where this is not optimal, inform the individual what you will be doing and check out that it is acceptable.
- **Personal priorities** – people with schizophrenia often know exactly what they want, and they want it now! Thus it might be necessary to restore a tooth first, even though this might not be optimal treatment planning, in order to engage the patient in other aspects of oral health/hygiene.
- **Perception** – it is prudent to ensure that you are always chaperoned and to keep detailed records as the individual with schizophrenia may have a different perception of an event from the reality.

An understanding dental team, aware of the issues associated with schizophrenia, with good patient management skills and an empathic attitude, may help to motivate a patient with schizophrenia towards good oral health.

2. Endogenous Depression

Endogenous depression results from a chemical imbalance in the brain, (e.g. a deficiency in the mood-enhancing chemical serotonin). One in 5 women and 1 in 15 men suffer from a bout of severe depression at least once in their lifetime. Many people will experience further episodes. Depression that coexists with learning disability and other mental illness can be difficult to diagnose or go undiagnosed, further complicating an already challenging situation.

Symptoms
Clinical depression is diagnosed when several of the following symptoms occur simultaneously for more than two weeks, with a marked effect on everyday life and the ability to function properly.

Typical symptoms of depression include:
- loss of appetite and weight loss, or comfort eating and weight gain
- tiredness and loss of concentration
- crying easily and feeling pessimistic
- loss of confidence and self-esteem and a sense of worthlessness
- mood swings
- difficulty in sleeping
- headaches
- suicidal thoughts.

Atypical facial pain occurs in approximately 10% of people with depression, and can be the presenting symptom. Interestingly 70% of people with atypical facial pain respond to treatment with antidepressants.

Management
Conventional treatment is with antidepressants. Dry mouth is amongst the side-effects of these drugs. Alternative approaches, such as low carbohydrate diets and natural remedies (including a derivative of amino acid methionine, St John's Wort and the B vitamins) are also used.

Oral Health
Like all people with long-standing mental illness, those with chronic depression are at risk of increased dental disease, and self-neglect. Xerostomic side-effects of antidepressant medication increase the risk of poor oral hygiene, periodontal disease and caries.

Dental Management
This requires patience and an empathic approach. People lose interest in life, not just oral hygiene. Where it is possible to enlist the help of a carer in maintaining oral hygiene, this is worthwhile.

3. Dementia

Dementia is a progressive, neurodegenerative disease that affects the ability to perform daily living activities. There are a number of types of both reversible and irreversible dementia. The commonest form is Alzheimer's disease (AD) accounting for 50–60% of dementias. It is one of the most protracted forms of dementia, thus, oral health is likely to be an issue at some stage during its process. The clinical features, symptoms and the principles applied to providing oral healthcare for people with AD and other types of dementia are similar, although the timescale of the dementia process may be different and in some cases accelerated, for example in CJD-related dementia.

Aetiology of AD
The immediate cause is the loss of neurones. Its aetiology is unknown, but a number of risk factors (including age, inherited family risk, brain damage, Down's syndrome and Herpes simplex) are recognised.

Onset of AD
This may be either early or, more commonly, late. Dementia currently affects over 750,000 people in the UK. Over 18,000 of them are under the age of 65. The prevalence rates are set out in Table 5-1.

Whilst the course the disease takes varies on an individual basis, the average life expectancy from diagnosis is 8 to 10 years. The commonest cause of death is infection.

Table 5-1 **Prevalence rates of dementia in the UK**

Age (years)	Prevalence
40-65	1 in 1000
65-70	1 in 50
70-80	1 in 20
80+	1 in 5

Diagnosis
Diagnosis is made over a period of time based on ruling out other types of dementia, recording symptoms, and the results of cognitive/memory tests. Confirmation of diagnosis can only be made at post mortem when specific pathology of senile plaques and neuro-fibrillary tangles are identified in the brain.

Clinical Features and Symptoms
AD is a progressive disease, appearing first as memory decline and, over several years, destroying cognition, personality, and ability to function. Con-

fusion and restlessness may also occur. Characteristic clinical features are memory loss, language deterioration, impaired visuospatial skills, poor judgement, indifferent attitude, but preserved motor function. The individual may also experience hallucinations and delusions. The type, severity, sequence, and progression of mental changes vary widely. Usually, AD is a slow disease, starting with mild memory problems and ending with severe brain damage.

Management
There is no cure for AD. Modern management is aimed at maintaining quality of life. Drugs can be used to help slow down its progression, and to control the associated depression, agitation and challenging behaviour. Many of these drugs have xerostomic side-effects.

Oral Health
Oral health is likely to decline as AD progresses. The impact of the disorder, especially in the latter stages, leads to poor oral hygiene with an increase in periodontal disease, higher levels of decay (both coronal and cervical) and a greater incidence of other dental problems such as denture wearing or the ability to comply with oral care. The xerostomic side-effects of prescribed medication contribute to these problems.

Oral Health Assessment
An oral health risk assessment that focuses on the individual's ability for self-care in oral hygiene and cooperation for treatment is essential at the point of diagnosis and throughout the progression of dementia. This allows the clinician to formulate appropriate oral care plans, preventive strategies and treatment options. Treatment planning needs to take account of:

- existing oro-dental disease
- current mouth care practices and preventive behaviour
- patterns of dental attendance
- dietary changes required to maintain nutritional health
- oral side-effects of medication
- communication
  - ability to express needs or wishes and to explain what is wanted
  - ability to understand and explain dental symptoms such as pain
- competence
  - ability to take part in the decision-making process about treatment
  - ability to give informed consent
  - ability to understand that oral hygiene needs to be carried out

- compliance
  - ability to perform daily living activities such as oral hygiene
  - ability to tolerate dental interventions
- carer support
  - with oral hygiene/preventive measures
  - to recognise, interpret and report behaviour change, which may indicate dental problems
  - to initiate oral care.

Expression of Oral Symptoms

Once a person is unable to interpret or vocalise pain or discomfort, changes in behaviour that can be indicative of oral pain include:
- refusal to eat (particularly hard or cold foods)
- constant pulling at the face
- increased drooling
- leaving previously worn dentures out of the mouth
- increased restlessness, moaning or shouting
- disturbed sleep
- refusal to cooperate with normal daily activities
- self-injurious behaviour
- aggressive behaviour towards carers.

General Principles for Oral Healthcare

When considering strategic, long-term oral care planning, the following guidelines are useful:
- Instigate appropriate preventive measures to minimise dental disease as soon as possible.
- Undertake dental intervention in the early stages of the condition to manage outstanding dental treatment needs.
- Ensure dentures are named, cleaned professionally on a regular basis, and renewed using a duplication technique when their replacement is necessary.
- Instigate regular reviews tailored to the individual's needs to maintain the oral status quo, avoid pain, and minimise further interventions.

On a day-to-day basis, the following guidelines are useful:
- Recognise that people have good and bad days. If possible, dental care is better postponed to a good day.
- Short attention spans mean the ability to cooperate is decreased; keep dental appointments within the individual's capacity to cope.
- Short-term memory loss means communication can become difficult and

tedious. Clear, short instructions repeated in the same words are useful. For example, "sit down" or "sit here" is much more likely to elicit the desired reaction than is the invitation to "please take a seat" or "would you like to sit down". The person with AD is likely to ask the same questions repeatedly; it is unhelpful to say "I have just told you ..." as this only adds to their sense of confusion. It is best to repeat the answer in the same words. Smiling and use of appropriate touch are useful, with reassuring gestures. Resist the temptation to raise your voice as shouting will not aid understanding.

• Emotional lability causes swings from laughing to crying within a short space of time. This is not as a result of dental treatment. It is a symptom of AD. Warning dental staff about the possibility of such mood swings makes it less distressing for them and easier to cope with.

Dental Treatment

The ability to comply with oral hygiene procedures and dental care is often influenced by past dental behaviour and experiences. People who have had regular dental treatment throughout their lives seem to remember what they are expected to do in the dental surgery and have little difficulty cooperating with simple procedures until the late stage of the disease. Dental management can be quite easy when dealing with a "happily confused", cooperative individual or even a passively compliant person. It can be very difficult, and sometimes impossible, when faced with someone who becomes distressed when interfered with in any way (e.g. washing, dressing, hair-brushing or tooth cleaning) or when a person is verbally and/or physically aggressive.

Determining the individual's level of social functioning and whether (s)he is physically or verbally abusive helps to determine the treatment modality that can be used. Treatment planning must also take account of the stage of the illness and the level of cognitive impairment. The dental index score described in Table 5-2 provides useful guidance on treatment planning approaches. The treatment philosophy should be based on the primary responsibility of the dentist to eliminate pain, control infection, and prevent new disease.

In the early stage (the first 4 years) of dementia most people can be treated in mainstream primary dental care services and most restorative and rehabilitative care is possible. Treatment should be planned, anticipating the person's decline in cooperation and ability for self-care. Key teeth can be identified (e.g. canines, molars, occluding pairs) and restored to function.

Restorative treatment should be high quality and low maintenance. Any advanced restorative treatment should only be planned in the knowledge that, when the individual can no longer provide oral self-care, a care-giver is prepared to take on this role. Rigorous preventive measures (both home- and surgery-based) should be put in place at this stage so that they become routine for both the individual and their carer.

In the moderate stage of the disease (2–8 years) a large proportion of people will still be able to be treated in mainstream primary dental services, although some people may require specialist care. During this stage the person is often

Table 5-2 **Assessment of ability to cooperate for dental treatment**

Can patient brush teeth or clean dentures?	Yes (0)	Needs some assistance (1)	Needs complete assistance (2)
Can patient verbalise chief complaint?	Yes (0)	To limited degree (1)	No (2)
Can patient follow simple instructions (e.g. sit in chair)?	Yes (0)	Occasionally complies (1)	Cannot follow instructions (2)
Can patient hold radiograph in mouth with film holder?	Yes (0)	Sometimes (1)	Never (2)
Is patient assaultive (bites/hits)?	No (0)	Sometimes (1)	Always (2)
Total score	0	5	10

Scoring system:
0-3 Mild disease (no change in treatment)
4-7 Moderate disease (modify treatment plan)
8-10 Severe disease (emergency treatment only)

Source: Niessen LC, Jones JA, Zocchi M, Gurian B. Dental care for the patient with Alzheimers's Disease. J Am Dent Ass 1985:110:207-209.

relatively physically healthy but has lost cognitive skills, and the focus of oral care changes from restorative and rehabilitative to maintenance and prevention. Some people are verbally and/or physically abusive at this stage, making treatment difficult. Sedation or general anaesthesia may be necessary for treatment. The decision will be based on the individual's ability to cooperate, their dental treatment needs, general health and social support. Rigorous prevention should be continued and more frequent recall visits and support for carers employed, as appropriate.

In the late stage of the disease (6–10 years) the person is more likely to require specialist care. They are severely cognitively impaired and often physically frail or disabled; they may be uncooperative, but no longer abusive or violent. Treatment at this stage focuses on prevention, maintaining oral comfort and emergency treatment. Familiar surroundings, routines and people are reassuring if a person is confused and in some instances domiciliary dental care can help cooperation enormously.

As dementia progresses, dental interventions should be kept as non-invasive as possible. For example, using Carisolv for caries removal, atraumatic restorative techniques (ART) with glass ionomer cement restorations, and regular application of chlorhexidine varnish to control root caries. If treatment beyond the individual's coping capacity is required, two questions need to be asked:
- Firstly, is the treatment necessary? If the answer to this question is yes, then the second question to ask is:
- How can it best be carried out?

The treatment planning then has to take account of the treatment modalities available, including a combination of oral or intranasal sedation with intravenous sedation, or general anaesthesia. The benefit of treatment has to be weighed up and at least balanced with the difficulties of providing it in terms of cooperation, consent, and restraint.

Consent

In situations where communication is questionable and the individual is considered not to have the capacity to give informed consent, it is prudent to involve family and/or carers in the decision-making process. In some residential settings a "best interests meeting" will be held, involving all parties, to decide whether the proposed dental treatment is in the best interests of the individual. Even when agreement is gained from relatives and carers, professional consent (that is two independent health care professionals agreeing that the treatment is in the best interests of the patient) should be sought in instances where proposed dental treatment is radical or irreversible.

Conclusions

- Mental illness is common.
- The majority of people with mental illness can be easily treated within mainstream primary dental care services.
- Whilst mental illness can impact on oral health, facial or oral symptoms can be the presenting signs of mental illness.

Further Reading

BSDH. Oral Healthcare for People with Mental Health Problems: Guidelines and Recommendations (2000). www.bsdh.org.uk

BSDH. Principles of Intervention for People Unable to Comply with Routine Dental Care (2006). www.bsdh.org.uk

Fiske J, Frenkel H, Griffiths J, Jones V. BSG/BSDH Guidelines for the Development of Local Standards of Oral Health Care for People with Dementia. Gerodontology 2006: Supplement 2.

Chapter 6

Managing Patients Who Require Antibiotic Cover

Aim

The aim of this chapter is to outline the reasons for prescribing antibiotic cover and to describe the most currently proposed regimes.

Outcome

After reading this chapter, the practitioner will be aware of the conditions and dental treatment that require antibiotic cover, the suggested regimes, and the current dilemmas surrounding antibiotic cover. The practitioner should be aware that guidelines change and they have a professional responsibility to keep up to date.

Introduction

The requirement for antibiotic cover (abc) is one of the more confusing areas in dentistry with different regimes adopted in different countries, in different areas of the UK or even between departments within the same hospital. National guidelines are produced by the Working Party of the British Society for Antimicrobial Chemotherapy (BSAC) and published in the Dental Practitioners' Formulary. The latest proposed UK guidelines have simplified recommended antibiotic cover regimes (Table 6-1).

In theory, the provision of antibiotic cover for dental treatment is linked to the prevention of infective endocarditis. However, there is a lack of any supporting evidence that dental treatment leads to infective endocarditis. A prospective double-blind trial is needed to evaluate the benefit of prophylactic antibiotics. This is unlikely to happen due to ethical considerations and the large numbers of people required to provide any significant findings.

Infective Endocarditis

Infective endocarditis carries a high risk of morbidity and mortality. Rapid diagnosis, effective treatment, and prompt recognition of complications

Table 6-1 **Prophylaxis for dental procedures** (continued over page)

High-risk cardiac factors requiring antibiotic prophylaxis	Previous infective endocarditis Cardiac valve replacement surgery, i.e. mechanical or biological prosthetic valves Surgically constructed systemic or pulmonary shunt or conduit
Dental procedures requiring antibiotic prophylaxis	All dental procedures involving dento-gingival manipulation
Antibiotic regimens for endocarditis prophylaxis	***All*** Preoperative mouth rinse with chlorhexidine gluconate 0.2% (10 ml for 1 minute) **No allergies** *Adults and children > 10 years* Amoxicillin 3 g orally one hour before dental procedure > 5 < 10 years of age 1.5 g < 5 years of age 750 mg **If allergic to penicillin** *Adults and children > 10 years* Clindamycin 600 mg orally one hour before dental procedure > 5 < 10 years of age 300 mg < 5 years of age 150 mg **Allergic to penicillin and unable to swallow capsules** *Adults and children > 10 years* Azithromycin 500 mg orally one hour before dental procedure > 5 < 10 years of age 300 mg < 5 years of age 200 mg

Table 6-1 **Prophylaxis for dental procedures** (continued)

Antibiotic regimens for endocarditis prophylaxis (continued)	**Intravenous regimens for dental treatment** (when considered expedient)
	Adults and children > 10 years A single IV dose of 1 g amoxicillin given just before the procedure or at induction of anaesthesia > 5 < 10 years of age 500 mg < 5 years of age 250 mg
	If allergic to penicillin *Adults and children > 10 years* A single IV dose of 300 mg clindamycin given at least 10 minutes before the procedure or at induction of anaesthesia > 5 < 10 years of age 150 mg < 5 years of age 75 mg
	Where a course of treatment involves several visits Visits should be at intervals of at least 14 days to allow healing of oral mucosal surfaces Where further dental procedures cannot be delayed, the antibiotic regimen should alternate between amoxicillin and clindamycin
	If allergic to penicillin Seek expert advice

Source: Gould FK, Elliott TSJ, Foweraker J, et al. Report of the Working Party of the British Society for Antimicrobial Chemotherapy: Guidelines for the Prevention of Endocarditis. J Antimicrob Chemother 2006;57:1035-1042.

are essential to good patient outcome. Appropriate action for its prevention in high-risk patients is paramount as infective endocarditis is an uncommon, but potentially fatal, infection of the endocardium or vascular endothelium. It has a reported incidence of 1500 cases a year in England and Wales and this is thought to be increasing due to:

- children with congenital heart disease surviving into adulthood
- an ageing population, with damaged hearts, surviving longer, and
- an increase in the number of intravenous drug users.

Infective endocarditis develops in vegetations formed on the valve leaflets or other sites on the endocardium where damage has occurred. The initial lesion is a platelet thrombus. Micro-organisms accumulate and multiply in the thrombus and more platelets and fibrin are deposited over the organisms. Eventually infective emboli break off to be deposited in different sites of the body. These septic emboli can cause gangrene of the fingers, stroke, myocardial infarction and pulmonary infarction. Other clinical features include fever, chronic renal failure and a new or changing heart murmur as the virulent organisms rapidly destroy the valve cusp producing ulceration and regurgitation.

Most commonly, infective endocarditis develops in valves which have been damaged due to rheumatic fever or congenital heart disease, but prosthetic valves can also be affected. Patient susceptibility to infective endocarditis is dependent on the underlying cardiac condition and the resulting changes to haemodynamic flow. The more severe the turbulence the more damage there is to the endothelium and the greater the risk of infective endocarditis. Small defects are more likely to cause turbulence than large ones, and surgically repaired atrial and ventricular septal defects are thought to be low risk. Patients who have had one episode of infective endocarditis are at increased risk of another episode.

Mortality varies depending on the infecting organism and is higher when a prosthetic valve is infected. Oral streptococci, and hence dental treatments, have been implicated in 47.5% of confirmed cases. Other commonly involved bacteria include enterococci and staphylococci, fungi and the haemophilus group. In intravenous drug users, where the risk arises from injecting drugs being made up with non-sterile water, more unusual micro-organisms such as *Candida*, *Aspergillus* and *Brucella* are involved.

Risk of Infective Endocarditis from Dental Treatment

Differing views have been held as to which cardiac conditions put patients undergoing invasive dental treatment at risk of developing infective endocarditis. The predisposing conditions and special risk patients are shown in Table 6-2.

There has been some debate about which dental treatments require antibiotic cover and whether the presence of bleeding is significant. It is now

Table 6-2 **Conditions predisposing to risk of infective endocarditis**

Conditions predisposing to infective endocarditis

- History of infective endocarditis
- Ventricular septal defect
- Patent ductus arteriosus
- Coarctation of the aorta
- Prosthetic heart valves
- Rheumatic and other acquired valvular disease
- Surgical constructed systemic-pulmonary shunts
- Persistent heart murmur
- Atrial septal defect repaired with a patch
- Hypotrophic cardiomyopathy

Patients not at risk from infective endocarditis

- After coronary bypass surgery
- Six months after surgery for:
  - Ligated ductus arteriosus
  - Surgically closed atrial or ventricular septal defects (without Dacron patch)
  - Isolated secundum atrial septal defect

Special risk patients

- Those with a previous history of infective endocarditis
- Those who require a general anaesthetic and have a prosthetic heart valve or are allergic to penicillin or who have had penicillin more than once in the previous month

Source: British National Formulary for Dentists, BSAC guidelines for antibiotic prophylaxis (1993).

thought that bleeding is not significant and some procedures, which produce little bleeding, can still cause a bacteraemia, for example, placement of rubber dam and matrix bands. The range of bacteraemias arising after different dental treatments is given in Table 6-3.

The emphasis on the cause of endocarditis has moved from procedure-related bacteraemia to cumulative bacteraemia. It has been postulated that "every-

Table 6-3 **Prevalence of bateraemia arising after various types of dental procedures and oral activity**

Procedure	Prevalence of bacteraemia
Extractions	
• Single	51%
• Multiple	68–100%
Periodontal surgery	
• Flap procedure	36–88%
• Gingivectomy	83%
Scaling and root planing	8–80%
Periodontal prophylaxis	0–40%
Endodontics	
• Intracanal intrumentation	0–31%
• Extracanal instrumentation	0–54%
Endodontic surgery	
• Flap reflection	83%
• Periapical curettage	33%
Toothbrushing	0–26%
Dental flossing	20–58%
Interproximal cleaning with toothpicks	20–40%
Irrigation devices	7–5%
Chewing	17–51%

Source: Seymour RA, Lowry J, Whitworth M, Martin MV. Infective endocarditis, dentistry and antibiotic prophylaxis; time for a rethink? Brit Dent J 2000;189:610-616.

day" bacteraemia is six million times greater than the bacteraemia from a single dental extraction, making it unlikely that dental procedures are solely responsible for causing infective endocarditis. Everyday procedures such as tooth brushing and chewing can cause bacteraemias that are significant to the risk of infective endocarditis and good oral health is more important than the provision of antibiotic cover.

As a result of this shift of view, the most currently proposed guidance recommends that the current practice of giving antibiotic cover to all patients with cardiac abnormalities is stopped. It explains that *antibiotic prophylaxis is only necessary for patients who have:*

- *a history of previous endocarditis*
- *had cardiac valve replacement surgery*
- *a surgically constructed systemic or pulmonary shunt or conduit.*

Another change of view is that antibiotic prophylaxis is now considered to prevent infective endocarditis by reducing bacterial adherence to damaged heart valves rather than by providing bactericidal blood levels. Removing bacteria after they have attached to valves may also be important and suggests that the timing of antibiotic cover should be reconsidered.

Risks from Using Antibiotics

An extreme view might be that all potentially at risk patients should be given cover for all dental care. However, this would result in many more cases of allergy, anaphylaxis and death. It would also contribute to the worldwide problem of the emergence of resistant strains of micro-organisms.

The medical and allergy history **must** always be updated before giving antibiotics and the dental team should be trained in the recognition and handling of allergic reactions, including anaphylaxis.

Care must be taken when prescribing antibiotics for patients who are taking other drugs; for example, the anticoagulant warfarin (the effect of which can be intensified) and oral contraceptives (the effect of which can be diminished). It is recommended that potential drug interactions are routinely checked before prescribing.

Antibiotic Cover and Dental Treatment

For high-risk patients the proposed new guidance recommends antibiotic cover is given for all dental procedures involving dentogingival manipulation or endodontics. A single oral dose of antibiotics is considered to provide adequate serum levels. On occasions the intravenous (IV) route of antibiotic administration may be appropriate and recommendations are given for antibiotic regimes using both oral and IV routes in Table 6-1.

Treatment Planning

The most important aspect of dental treatment for people at risk of infective endocarditis is good oral hygiene through tailored preventive advice; delivery of high-quality dental care; and monitoring through regular recalls. Where invasive treatment is required, careful planning can minimise the frequency of use of antibiotic prophylaxis. This approach has the twofold benefit of reducing the likelihood of development of antibiotic resistant strains and of allergy.

Both the current UK BSAC and the proposed guidelines recommend the use of chlorhexidine mouthwash before dental care in order to reduce numbers of oral bacteria (by around 95%) and reduce the intensity of any bacteraemia related to treatment. Direct irrigation of periodontal pockets is not recommended as this can, itself, cause a bacteraemia.

Local Anaesthesia

Intraligamentary anaesthesia carries the risk of a high load bacteraemia and should be avoided in "at risk" patients. For those patients taking warfarin, and for whom nerve blocks may carry a risk of bleeding and haematoma formation, alternative methods should be considered such as infiltration with articaine, which is thought to have better bony absorption than lignocaine.

Restorative Dentistry

Full mouth pocket charting should be combined with scaling and antibiotic prophylaxis given once, rather than on two separate occasions. Also, it is prudent to do half mouth root planing over a longer appointment rather than quadrant by quadrant debridement. At present all professional cleaning procedures except air polishing require cover. There have been documented cases of infective endocarditis following what was described as minimal supragingival scaling which have resulted in medicolegal claims. It is unwise to carry out any scaling procedure without antibiotic cover, as it is impossible to guarantee that trauma to the gingival margin will not occur. The latest proposals clarify previous areas of confusion around the need, or not, to provide antibiotic cover for procedures such as the placement of a matrix band, and gingival retraction cord below the dento-epithelial junction. This is now necessary for high-risk patients. The use of chlorhexidine mouthwash before restorative procedures is still recommended.

Longer appointments, needed to maximise invasive treatment under each episode of abc, can be difficult for anxious patients and recourse to the use of conscious sedation or general anaesthesia for these patients should be considered.

Endodontic Treatment
The draft BSAC guidance recommends abc for all endodontic treatment including pulpotomies in the primary dentition, once again removing areas of confusion.

Paediatric Dentistry
For the "at risk" child requiring multiple dental procedures, an argument can be made for all treatment to be carried out in one visit under general anaesthesia.

Dental Treatment and Heart Surgery

People due to receive intracardiac valves, conduits or grafts should be referred for dental assessment and treatment prior to cardiac surgery. Ideally, oral hygiene should be optimised and any dental interventions carried out at least 14 days prior to surgery to allow for mucosal healing. This is not possible in emergency situations and in these situations a dental risk assessment should be undertaken as soon as is practicable following surgery. Elective dental procedures should be delayed until at least three months after cardiac surgery.

Dental Treatment and Prosthetic Implants

Whilst it is theoretically possible that a bacteraemia during dental care could cause infection of an implanted prosthetic device, there is no evidence that prophylaxis is required for people with breast implants, pacemakers, intraocular lenses or prosthetic vascular devices. It has been suggested that people with hydrocephalus shunts do require cover. There are two types of shunts used to remove excess cerebrospinal fluid from the brain in hydrocephaly: ventriculo-atrial (VA), where the CSF is taken to the heart via the internal jugular vein; and ventriculo-peritoneal (VP), which shunts the CSF into the abdominal cavity. Most shunt infections occur within two months of placement and are due to skin or airborne organisms. Oral flora have been found in a very small number of shunt infections.

There have been no randomised controlled trials concerning the use of antibiotic prophylaxis but the risk appears to be almost negligible for patients with either a VA or a VP shunt and current guidance from the North West Medicines Information Centre is that people with VA or VP shunts do not require abc.

Dental Treatment and Joint Replacements

Prophylaxis for people with prosthetic joints remains a controversial area. Anxieties occur because late infection of a total hip replacement can require its total removal, debridement and prolonged antibiotic therapy. It has not been established how frequently, or even if, dental interventions are responsible for such infections and current BSAC guidelines do not recommend antibiotic cover for patients with joint replacements. While it would be easy for dentists to delegate responsibility to the surgeon this is not appropriate. If a surgeon insists on antibiotic cover, they should be referred to the guidelines for dentists in the British National Formulary. If there is concern about the risk of bacteraemia from dental procedures, chlorhexidine mouthwash can be used one to two minutes before treatment.

In 2003 the American Dental Association and the American Academy of Orthopaedic Surgeons published an advisory statement that, on the whole, antibiotic cover is not indicated for dental patients with total hip replacements. However, it pointed out that in a few high-risk groups antibiotics should be considered. People with rheumatoid arthritis, where there does seem to be an increased susceptibility to haematogenous infection, are considered at high risk. Whilst an argument has been made for antibiotic cover for people with diabetes, haemophilia and those on long-term steroid therapy, the evidence is not convincing and antibiotic cover is not routinely recommended.

Medicolegal Considerations

Aside from the clinical need for antibiotic cover, consideration must be given to the medicolegal aspects. One retrospective study found 53 cases where infective endocarditis followed dental care with only one instance where appropriate antibiotic cover had been given at the right time. In many cases inappropriate antibiotics had been given and medical histories were found to be incomplete, out of date, or not taken.

For all patients requiring the provision of antibiotic prophylaxis the following should be recorded in their notes:
- cardiac risk for infective endocarditis
- the type and dose of antibiotic chosen
- the absence of allergy to the chosen drug
- time of administration of drug
- the dental procedure undertaken

- time dental procedure commenced
- post-operative instructions given to the patient regarding illness/fever post-operatively, for example warned to seek immediate medical attention if (s)he develops a high fever within 10 days of receipt of the dental treatment, and
- preventive advice given.

Conclusions

- Prophylaxis is often thought to refer to the provision of antibiotic cover. It should be thought of more broadly as the maintenance of good oral hygiene and prevention of oral disease to reduce the frequency and load of bacteraemias caused by chewing and tooth brushing and to reduce the need for invasive dental treatment.
- Patients should understand that their day-to-day oral hygiene measures are more important than professional treatment and taking antibiotics.
- Proposed latest guidance restricts antibiotic prophylaxis to high-risk groups; extends antibiotic cover to all dental procedures involving dentogingival manipulation and endodontics; and recommends oral delivery of antibiotics unless IV delivery is considered expedient.

Further Reading

Gould FK, Elliott TSJ, Foweraker J, et al. Report of the Working Party of the British Society for Antimicrobial Chemotherapy: Guidelines for the Prevention of Endocarditis. J Antimicrob Chemother 2006;57:1035-1042.

Seymour RA. Lowry J, Whitworth M, Martin MV. Infective endocarditis, dentistry and antibiotic prophylaxis; time for a rethink? Br Dent J 2000;189:610-616.

Chapter 7
Managing Immunocompromised Patients

Aim

The aim of this chapter is to describe the oral health problems that immuno-compromised patients may present with and how to effectively plan treatment for this group.

Outcome

After reading this chapter you should be able to recognise the conditions that may lead to immunosuppression and those patients that are at risk, i.e. immuno-compromised in relation to oral healthcare. You should be able to assess the preventive and prophylactic regimes that may be necessary to carry out a range of dental treatments, and longer-term care, for immunocompromised patients.

Introduction

Immunodeficient, *immunosuppressed* and *immunocompromised* are the common terms used to refer to patients whose immune system is not functioning optimally. In the context of this chapter:

- *Immunodeficient* describes any state where the immune system is functioning below the optimum level.
- *Immunosuppression* refers to artificially depressed immune systems; for example, caused by drugs used to control disease processes or prevent rejection of transplanted organs.
- *Immunocompromised* describes patients with a medical condition where their immune function is inherently poor, suppressed artificially or depressed due to illness and where they may be at significant risk of concurrent illness due to the reduced immune function.

The term "immunocompromised" has the most clinical relevance, indicating that the risks of any complications may be increased as a result of dental treatment. As immunocompromised, patients may have significantly reduced ability to cope with dental treatment. It is important to be able to recognise this group of patients and to have strategies in place that take account of their medical condition during dental treatment.

Immunocompromised patients can present with oral signs of poor immune function and be at risk of other conditions, with or without oral manifestations. For example, Kaposi's sarcoma and pneumocystis carinii pneumonia in patients with HIV disease.

Conditions Leading to Immunodeficiency

There are many medical texts that describe the underlying histological faults that lead to the different types of immunodeficiency. The reader is referred to such texts for information on the pathological processes involved. However, in order to understand the clinical relevance of immunodeficiency some explanation of taxonomy is required as this relates to cause and presentation.

The simplest classification is to divide the causes into:
- innate or primary (congenital, genetic, internal or inherent)
- acquired or secondary (environmental or external) conditions.

Innate (Primary) Immunodeficiency States
Genetic immunodeficiency states are relatively uncommon and can be sex-linked or autosomal in inheritance. Defects can occur in any or all of the white cell lines and/or the complement system producing very variable clinical effects. For example in 2 X-linked conditions presentation can be quite different, in Wiskott-Aldrich syndrome there is deficient production of IgM and in Bruton's disease any or all of the immunoglobulins may be deficient.

In Common Variable Immunodeficiency (CVID) there can be deficiencies in both B and T cell production resulting in defects in both "arms" of the immune system. In some cases cell numbers are normal, but cell maturation or production defects exist. Finally, a number of these conditions have defects in other blood cell lines, such as platelets resulting in clotting defects as well as issues relating to infection and healing.

The terminology can be confusing. In the conditions cited in Table 7-1, the immune deficiency is the primary or innate disease. There are other innate diseases that have "secondary" immunodeficiencies. Insulin-dependent diabetes mellitus and Down's syndrome are two examples where the subject has an innate condition, of which immunodeficiency may be a part, but the immunodeficiency is not generally the main presenting feature.

Immunodeficiency in these conditions can be variable, ranging from insignificant (rendering it clinically imperceptible) to severe enough to pro-

Table 7-1 **Innate (primary) immunodeficiency states**

Agammaglobulinaemia

Hypogammaglobulinaemia

Bruton's Disease – X-linked agammaglobulinaemia (XLA)

Common Variable Immunodeficiency (CVID)

Severe Combined Immunodeficiency (SCID)

Good's Syndrome – thymoma and B & T cell immunodeficiency

Wiskott-Aldrich Syndrome – hypoimmunoglobulinaemia M and thrombocytopenia

Selective IgA deficiency

Selective IgG sub-class deficiencies

Duncan's Syndrome – X-linked Lymphoproliferative Syndrome (XLP)

C1 esterase inhibitor deficiency – hereditary angioedema

Job Syndrome – hyperimmunoglobulin E Syndrome

---

duce "primary" symptoms. An example of the latter is the tendency towards advanced periodontal disease in people with diabetes and Down's syndrome. The immunodeficiency is not "secondary" to the primary condition *per se*, but is intrinsically part of the condition.

Acquired (Secondary) Immunodeficiency States

A number of conditions can cause immunodeficiency. The classes of conditions that may exhibit immunodeficiency are:
- infectious diseases, e.g. HIV disease
- malignancies, e.g. Hodgkin's disease and the leukaemias
- autoimmune diseases, e.g. systemic lupus erythematosus, rheumatoid arthritis
- nutritional deficiencies, e.g. iron and vitamin deficiencies
- other miscellaneous conditions, e.g. sickle cell disease, can lead to splenic hypofunction which in turn can lead to immunodeficiency; idiopathic thrombocytopaenic purpura may require splenectomy leading to immunodeficiency
- iatrogenic suppression (e.g. antirejection drug therapy) for solid (e.g. heart, kidney and liver) and non-solid (e.g. bone marrow) organ transplantation; auto-immune diseases, such as systemic lupus erythematosus, requiring drug-induced immune suppression as part of their management; some

tumours and the leukaemias respond to immunosuppressive drug regimes. Drugs used include azathioprine, cyclosporin, tacrolimus and mycophenylate.

The internet has revolutionised the ability of patients and clinicians to access information relating to medical conditions such as these and it can be easily accessed as a first point of reference.

White Blood Cell Count

A total white blood cell (WBC) count ranges between 4500 and 10,000 cells/microl. A WBC count below 4500 is immune depressed and, as a rule of thumb, a leucopoenia below 2000 (2×10^9/l) renders the patient immunocompromised and at possible risk of infection. Less than 500 (5×10^9/l) would make them susceptible to fatal infection.

The differential WBC count must also be borne in mind (Table 7-2). It should always add up to 100% for each patient. A normal total count combined with a disproportionate differential complicates the picture and may still put the patient at risk. For example, a count of 5000 u/l is in the normal range but the differential may show the percentage of lymphocytes at only 2%. This is an agranulocytosis and the patient is at risk of infection.

The functional status of the cells must also be considered as this can be low despite adequate numbers. Cell function can only be assessed by specialist tests and is the realm of specialist immunology or haematology departments.

Assessing Immunodeficiency in Relation to Oral Healthcare

If a patient presents with a condition exhibiting immunodeficiency you need to:
• Know whether the severity of the condition is relevant to the proposed dental treatment.
• Be aware of any oral conditions that may become evident due to the reduced immune function. HIV disease is an example of this and the reader is directed to texts available on this topic.
• Be aware that during the history and examination process any sign of oral ulceration or other mucosal irregularity, bacterial or fungal overgrowth, unexplained tissue swelling or dysfunction may be related to the immunodeficiency.

Table 7-2 **White cell differentials**

White cell type	Count
Lymphocytes	$1.3–3.5 \times 10^9/l$ (approximately 20–40% of the white blood count). Decreased counts are seen following chemotherapy and whole-body radiotherapy and during steroid therapy, bone marrow diseases and systemic lupus erythematosus. HIV disease counts measure CD4 and CD8 T-lymphocytes. The CD4 normal range is approximately $500–1500/mm^3$. The CD8 normal range is approximately $230–750/mm^3$ with a CD4/CD8 ratio of 1.2–3.8.
Neutrophils	$2.0–7.5 \times 10^9/l$ (approximately 40–70% of the white blood count). Decreased counts occur with infections such as viral, TB, brucellosis and typhoid. Drug-induced neutropenia is seen with carbimazole, chloramphenicol, phenytoin and the sulphonamides. Neutropenia is also seen in B_{12} or folate deficiency, rheumatoid arthritis, splenic hyperfunction and systemic lupus erythematosus.
Monocytes	$0.2–0.8 \times 10^9/l$ (approximately 2–10% of the white blood count).
Eosinophils	$0.04–0.44 \times 10^9/l$ (approximately 1–5% of the white blood count).
Basophils	$0–0.1 \times 10^9/l$ (approximately 0–1% of the white blood count)

Liaison with the patient's medical specialist(s) is paramount for obtaining copies of recent serial full blood counts, white cell differentials and function tests, thus allowing you to determine the amount and timing of any proposed dental treatment. Whilst a single white cell count can be useful, it only provides a "snapshot" view and serial counts give a fuller picture of trends in the condition. Remember that differential counts do not give any indication of function. The total number of cells may be normal, but if they have very low function then the numbers are irrelevant. This is where liaison with the specialists in immunology and haematology becomes vital.

What Do You Do When Faced with an Immunocompromised Patient?

Liaison

The first principle is to take a full history from the patient and contact the patient's specialist(s). They may have specific recommendations that need to be taken into account for the patient's dental treatment. For example, patients with CVID may be receiving intravenous immunoglobulins at set regular intervals and dental treatment is best timed to follow shortly after a set of injections when the immune status will be at its best. Patients undergoing chemotherapy will have specific "rest periods" during their drug treatments and so may have times when dental treatment is best scheduled.

Certain specialist units may have specific local protocols for treatment timing and antibiotic prophylaxis prior to dental treatment in immuno-compromised patients. Whilst patients may inform you of them, it is always worth checking directly with the relevant specialist unit. For instance, they may advise avoidance of all elective dental treatment in the three months following a transplant, so that immunosuppressive drug regimes can be established, with treatment in the three- to six-month period undertaken only on their advice.

Check Patient Factors

Patients may require specific prophylactic measures due to their disease. For example, patients who have had a splenectomy to help idiopathic thrombo-cytopenic purpura are advised to be immunised against meningococcus, haemophilic influenza b and pneumococcus and many take prophylactic low-dose penicillin for some years following surgery. Patients with HIV infection have regular CD4 and viral load counts and checking with them and their general or specialist medical practitioners allows assessment of the condition and its relevance to dental care to be made.

Oral Hygiene and Risk

It is important to ensure that the patient's oral hygiene is of the highest order and that the patient understands the importance of any oral infections in relation to their general condition. Try to reduce the risks of mucogingival infections through patient education and motivation. Treat local infections rigorously using topical and systemic agents as required. Good mechanical cleaning, short-term use of chlorhexidine mouthwashes and systemic antibiotics are the mainstay of treatment here.

The patient may feel that such issues come low down in their list of priorities but it is incumbent on all dental professionals to ensure that patients understand their importance.

Infection Control

One of the main ways to minimise the risk of infection from dental treatment is to ensure that all dental unit water lines are thoroughly flushed and cleaned prior to treating immunocompromised patients. Dental unit water lines that stand unused for any length of time can develop high levels of bacterial "colony forming units" (CFUs) in the water tubing. The use of high-speed handpieces may then deliver this in an aerosol form to the patient. Rigorous pre-use flushing is known to reduce this risk. Concomitantly the use of high-volume suction will reduce the chance of inhaling dental handpiece aerosol spray. The use of a rubber dam is also highly recommended to cut down aerosol inhalation.

Treat the Symptoms

Patients on immunosuppressant therapy or with immunodeficiency states can suffer from several painful oral conditions. Oral ulceration, mucositis, burning mouth and xerostomia are not uncommon. Oral infections, (bacterial, viral and fungal) may occur and healing following surgical treatment may be prolonged. Rigorous treatment of oral infections is necessary. Pain control is vital and care must be taken to ensure adequate pain control is built into the patient's treatment plan. Many mouthwashes can be irritating to patients and may need to be "watered-down" to allow use and improve compliance. Rinses containing alcohol should be avoided as they cause stinging. Holding ice chips in the mouth immediately prior to treatment has been reported to help chemotherapy patients cope with pain from mucositis.

Artificial saliva can be helpful for patients with xerostomia, although, many patients find using frequent sips of cool water just as beneficial. Fluoride rinses are valuable in preventing caries, and diet advice (with information about sugar frequency and caries) is important. Oral hygiene advice may need to include the use of a soft toothbrush to avoid gingival trauma.

Prophylaxis for Dental Treatment

Immunocompromised patients are susceptible to infection from a wide range of micro-organisms and may be at risk of operatively-induced bacteraemia and post-operative infection. They may also be taking medication for their medical condition that requires prophylaxis in dentistry (e.g. corticosteroids). In patients taking oral steroid therapy of over 10 mg/day, preoperative steroid supplementation can be carried out using standard regimes. Current guidance favours oral dose-doubling regimes or low doses (25 mg) of intravenous hydrocortisone for routine dental procedures requiring cover.

The indications and drug regimes for antibiotic prophylaxis in immunocompromised patients are not the same as those for the prophylaxis of cardiac conditions although, in practice, similar regimes are often used. There is a degree of variation in the types and dosages of prophylaxis used and the treatments requiring cover. This depends upon variables related to the patient's medical condition. For example, a patient who is receiving chemotherapy for chronic leukaemia will have different risk variables to someone who is having immunosuppressive therapy for rheumatoid arthritis and has multiple joint replacements; or to someone having whole body irradiation and bone marrow transplantation.

The dental reason for providing prophylaxis may warrant a different type of cover. For example, an immunosuppressed patient at risk of lung infection from a full-mouth ultrasonic scale may be covered with a single dose regime similar to that provided for prevention of endocarditis. Whereas, a patient who is immunocompromised due to chemotherapy, and is undergoing the surgical removal of a molar, may require cover for longer to facilitate postoperative healing. This may warrant a regime similar to that given for cover in those patients at risk of osteoradionecrosis (see Chapter 8) with oral antibiotics given for a number of weeks post-operatively.

In patients with haematological dyscrasias, such as low platelet counts, liaison with the patient's haematologist will allow decisions to be made on whether haematological cover, such as platelet infusion, is required.

As guidelines change with improved knowledge, it is not the intention in this chapter to be prescriptive and produce fixed antibiotic prophylaxis regimes for all possibilities, but to point out the importance of being aware of the clinical conditions and situations that may require antibiotic prophylaxis. You can then discuss and arrange the individual regime for the patient, according to need, with their specialist(s).

Plan the Dental Treatment around the Condition
Whether the treatment required is preventive, restorative or surgical:
• Plan the treatment around the patient's condition taking account of the variables already described.
• Link the requirements and requests of the patient's medical specialists into the treatment planning process.
• Ensure that the patient understands the necessity for you to consult widely and that this can prolong the time taken to complete treatment, thus helping to avoid complaints borne out of impatience.
• Arrange any preoperative blood tests and allot time for pre-treatment prophylaxis.

Follow-up
Ensure thorough follow-up, in particular when surgical treatment is planned, as healing can be slow and infection risks remain for longer. General oral health review intervals should be shorter than for the general population, as rapid progression of dental disease can be a feature of being immunocompromised. Hence, oral health surveillance is important in this group of people to allow early detection of problems and early implementation of preventive and treatment strategies.

Conclusions

• Immunocompromised patients may be at risk of a number of complications from dental treatment.
• Recognising the signs of an immunocompromised patient through good history and examination processes and consultation with their specialist(s) is vitally important if operative and post-operative problems are to be avoided.
• Clinical monitoring and surveillance in this group should be rigorous, with follow-up maintained over longer than normal periods as immunocompromised patients can exhibit higher levels of oral health problems and complications than in the general population.

Further Reading

Little JW, Falace DA, Miller CS, Rhodus NL. Dental Management of the Medically Compromised Patient (5th edn). St Louis, Missouri: Mosby, 1997.

Chapter 8
Managing the Patient Having Radiotherapy

Aim

The aim of this chapter is to describe the changes caused by radiotherapy to the head and neck region and the relevance of these changes to oral health.

Outcome

After reading this chapter you will understand the factors that need to be taken into account when managing patients who will be having, or who have had, radiotherapy affecting the head and neck region.

Introduction

The dental practitioner may be the first to notice cancers of the lip, tongue, mouth and pharynx. In the UK, for example, about 4400 new cancer cases occur in these areas each year, as well as other cancers in the head and neck region (Table 8-1).

Facts about oral cancer include:
- the number of cases increased by 19% between 1995 and 2001
- mortality remains high and has changed little in the last 30 years
- over 90% are squamous cell carcinoma
- there is a higher incidence in men, but it is increasing in women (ratio < 2:1)
- occurs mainly in people aged > 50 years, but is increasing in younger people
- 25% of people develop a second primary cancer within three years
- early detection and treatment improves survival rate and treatment can be less aggressive with a better cosmetic and functional outcome
- lip cancer has the best outcome with a 90% five-year survival
- early-stage mouth cancers have a 60–90% five-year survival rate, but for late presentation the five-year survival rate is 30%
- in general the survival rate is less for tumours that are more posterior and less accessible
- survival is better in younger patients and more affluent people.

Table 8-1 **Head and neck cancers – UK 2001**

Site	New registrations
Lip	359
Tongue	1239
Mouth	1404
Pharynx	1168
Other parts of oral cavity	230
Salivary glands	526
Nasopharynx	223
Larynx	2407

Source: Office for National Statistics

Contributing factors to 80% of cases of oral cancer in developed countries are tobacco use and excess alcohol consumption. The risk associated with smoking is dose and duration related. Cessation leads to a fall in risk and after 10 years the risk is the same as for non-smokers. Other risk factors are outlined in Table 8-2. Increases in smoking and alcohol consumption are the likely reason for the increased incidence of oral cancer in under

Table 8-2 **Risk factors in oral cancer**

Predisposing factors	Potentially malignant conditions
Tobacco – smoked or chewed	Leucoplakia
Alcohol	Erythroplakia
Betel use (includes areca nut)	Submucous fibrosis
Low fruit and vegetable diet	Erosive lichen planus
Sun exposure to lower lip	Immunosuppression (e.g. transplant patients)
Viruses (e.g. human papilloma virus)	
First-degree relative affected	

45-year-olds. However, around 25% of younger patients who develop oral cancer, in particular women, have not been exposed to the known major risk factors.

Early treatment of oral cancer achieves better outcome with longer survival time and improved quality of life. Whilst population screening would not be cost-effective, dentists have the opportunity to screen their patients. Those with risk factors should be identified and given appropriate preventive advice. Those with suspicious lesions or premalignant conditions should be referred urgently to a specialist unit for investigation.

Treatment options depend on the stage of the tumour and include surgery, radiotherapy, surgery with post-operative radiotherapy, and radiotherapy with chemotherapy. Surgery and radiotherapy are equally effective in treating early disease, but surgery and post-operative radiotherapy give a better survival time in later disease. The aim of surgery is to remove the primary tumour, with an adequate tissue margin. Its use is appropriate where the tumour is accessible, large, invading bone and when the medical risk of an operation is acceptable. Radiotherapy is generally used for small tumours, inaccessible sites, and patients with poor risk for general anaesthesia. It may be used following surgery when there is a narrow excision margin, or to the neck where there is extracapsular spread from the lymph nodes. The advantages and disadvantages of surgery and radiotherapy are outlined in Table 8-3.

Radiotherapy

Radiotherapy is the use of ionising radiation to treat disease by damaging the cellular DNA. The radiation can be X-ray beams produced by high-energy electrons hitting an appropriate target or gamma radiation produced by decay of radioactive isotopes. External beam radiation with electrons produced in a linear accelerator is most commonly used in the head and neck region. Interstitial brachytherapy (placement of a radioactive source, usually iridium, in the tumour area) can be used in the mouth for small tumours. It causes fewer side-effects but requires special nursing procedures during treatment. Accurate positioning of radiation beams, confined to the tumour area, is important to ensure unwanted side-effects are minimised. To assist this, the area is immobilised during treatment through the use of a plastic head shell or mask worn by the patient and fixed to the treatment couch (see Fig 8-1). The actual radiotherapy treatment takes less than a minute in each field.

Table 8-3 **Advantages and disadvantages of surgery and radiotherapy**

	Surgery	**Radiotherapy**
Advantages	Extent of tumour can be seen and tumour removed More tissue available for histopathology	General anaesthesia not needed Preserves speech and swallowing Preserves appearance
Disadvantages	Perioperative mortality and morbidity Anaesthesia/paraesthesia Deformity Speech impairment Eating problems Social problems Psychological problems	Oral side-effects – Mucositis – Dry mouth – Loss of taste – Trismus – Caries – Risk of osteoradionecrosis

The unit of radiation dose is the Gray (Gy) which is a measure of absorbed energy (1 Gy = 1J/kg). Radiation schedules vary, but are typically 50–65 Gy divided into fractions over four to six weeks.

Adjuvant chemotherapy may be used with radiotherapy, depending on the tumour type, to decrease the local recurrence rate. At the present time fluorouracil and cisplatin are used. Palliative radiotherapy, lower dose and shorter duration, may be used for incurable cancers to reduce pain and to improve quality of life.

Effects of Radiotherapy in the Head and Neck Region

Radiotherapy causes both short- and longer-term general and oral side-effects (Table 8-4). One of the key recommendations of the National Institute of Clinical Excellence (NICE) is the need to provide a complete service from pretreatment assessment to rehabilitation to improve patient care and quality of life. This requires careful treatment planning. Generally, the multidisciplinary oncology team includes a restorative dentist who is responsible for coordinating the patient's dental care before, dur-

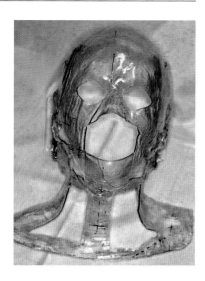

Fig 8-1 Mask for consistent positioning during radiotherapy.

ing and after treatment. This may well be in liaison with the patient's general dental practitioner.

Oral Assessment Prior to Radiotherapy

All patients having radiotherapy to the head and neck region should have an oral assessment prior to its commencement. This is a busy and anxious time for patients and their families and it is important that they see dental care as

Table 8-4 **Side-effects of radiotherapy**

During radiotherapy		Longer term
Oral effects	**General effects**	**Oral effects**
Mucositis	Fatigue	Caries
Dry mouth	Weight loss	Periodontal disease
Taste alteration	Skin burns	Osteoradionecrosis
Oral flora changes	Blood changes with full-body radiotherapy	*In childhood:*
Tooth hypersensitivity		Impaired facial growth
Trismus		Dental abnormalities

a part of improving their outcome. As well as a clinical assessment, a radiographic assessment is necessary to fully assess every tooth and its surrounding structures, and to look for buried roots or unerupted teeth that may have associated pathology.

Because of the associated risk of developing osteoradionecrosis from an infected tooth or extraction site following radiotherapy, the prognosis of every tooth must be considered carefully. It is not always possible to predict prognosis, but oral hygiene and caries rate are useful prognostic indicators in planning dental treatment. When assessing teeth regarding extraction prior to radiotherapy the following factors should be considered:

- general oral hygiene status
- caries rate
- extent of decay/risk of restoration failure of each tooth
- periodontal status and prognosis of each tooth
- endodontic status and prognosis of each tooth
- position of the tooth in relation to the radiotherapy
- whether it is a mandibular or maxillary tooth
- difficulty of extraction, should it be necessary in future
- whether it is a strategic tooth in terms of aesthetics or function.

Patients need to be highly motivated to maintain good oral hygiene during radiotherapy when their mouths are sore. If oral hygiene deteriorates it is likely that caries and periodontal disease will develop rapidly.

Partial and complete dentures should be assessed for fit and if they are causing trauma or have any sharp edges should be adjusted. If dentures are comfortable they should be worn during the course of radiotherapy to help eating, as it may be difficult to readjust to them later. A sore, dry mouth may make denture wear difficult. Denture hygiene needs to be impeccable to help reduce *Candida* infection.

Treatment Prior to Radiotherapy

It is ideal to complete all dental treatment before radiotherapy starts. Routine restorations can be carried out afterwards provided the prognosis of the tooth is not in doubt. Impressions may be taken to construct mouthguards or for obturator planning. Upper and lower mouthguards worn during radiotherapy reduce radiation scatter from metallic restorations and subsequent soft tissue damage and soreness (Fig 8-2). The trays can be used later for fluoride gel application.

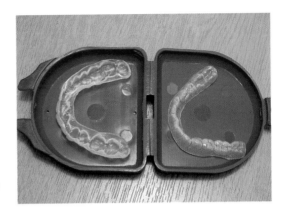

Fig 8-2 Tooth shields for use during radiotherapy.

Planned extractions should be carried out as soon as possible, with a minimum of seven days before the commencement of radiotherapy, to allow optimal healing. It is advisable to give a course of antibiotics post-extraction. Occasionally, multiple or complex extractions make it necessary to delay the start of radiotherapy. In addition, a full mouth scaling should be carried out and advice given on care of the mouth during radiotherapy. It is difficult for patients to assimilate all the information and an advice leaflet that the patient can refer to is essential. Patients should be encouraged to contact the dentist at any time if they have problems.

Children should be seen by a paedodontist who can monitor facial growth and dental development which may be affected by radiotherapy. Any teeth that are within three months of exfoliation or have caries close to the pulp should be extracted prior to radiotherapy. Orthodontic treatment should be discontinued.

Oral Management During Radiotherapy
There are a number of factors that can affect oral status, and which need to be considered during radiotherapy:

1. Dry Mouth
Xerostomia and altered salivary composition can occur within a day of starting radiotherapy. Residual saliva is thick and viscous and may form unpleasant lumps requiring the use of hydrogen peroxide mouthwash or suction for removal. Reduced saliva leads to difficulty chewing, swallowing, carrying out oral hygiene and wearing dentures; loss of taste; hypersensitivity; changes in the oral flora; and increased caries risk. Patients should be advised to:

- avoid sweets or sweet/acidic drinks to alleviate symptoms
- sip water or use a recommended saliva substitute
- use a high fluoride toothpaste (bought over the counter or prescribed)
- use Vaseline on dry lips, especially at night.

There may be improvements in salivary gland function up to two years after radiotherapy, but for some patients the function never returns and they have permanent xerostomia. Reservoirs that hold artificial saliva have been successfully incorporated into dentures.

2. Mucositis

Mucositis is an early and painful side-effect of radiotherapy treatment. It is caused by decreased mitosis so that the mucosa becomes thin, inflamed and ulcerated with a yellow covering (Fig 8-3). The inflammation starts 12–15 days into radiotherapy and usually resolves within a few weeks of completion of treatment. It makes eating and speaking very difficult. Advice to alleviate sore mouth includes:

- rinsing with soluble paracetamol 45 minutes before eating, or using Difflam immediately before eating
- 2% lidocaine mouthwash may also be prescribed
- avoiding spicy food, smoking and alcohol.

3. Loss of taste

Damage to the taste buds and lack of saliva cause alteration in taste, making food less palatable. Taste usually returns after a few months, but there may be some permanent loss after high doses of irradiation.

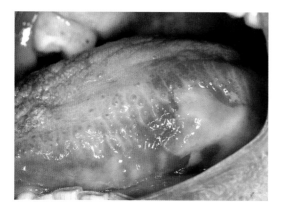

Fig 8-3 Radiation-induced mucositis.

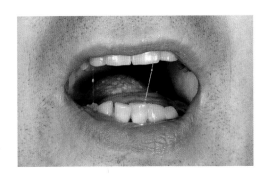

Fig 8-4 Trismus after radiotherapy.

4. Oral flora changes

With reduced buffering and antibacterial action of saliva there is a shift in oral flora with increased numbers of *Candida* and the cariogenic organisms *Streptococcus mutans* and *Lactobacillus*. These changes start within two weeks of commencing radiotherapy and continue after its completion. *Candida* should be treated with antifungals such as nystatin sugar-free suspension, miconazole gel or fluconazole suspension.

5. Trismus

Fibrosis of the masticatory muscles and reduction in their blood supply may cause trismus during radiotherapy, or up to six months afterwards, and can be permanent. This makes eating, oral hygiene and the provision of dental care difficult (Fig 8-4). Patients should be advised to carry out gentle jaw exercises to avoid trismus developing.

6. General oral hygiene

This is complicated by xerostomia and mucositis. Brushing should be carried out if possible, but may require use of a soft brush or even an oral swab dipped in chlorhexidine if too sore or for difficult areas (Fig 8-5). The use of chlorhexidine mouthwash (10 ml x 0.2% twice daily) is recommended. Its use should start two weeks prior to radiotherapy and be continued until effective brushing is possible. The taste may be too strong in which case it can be diluted with an equal quantity of water. Also, patients should be warned about extrinsic staining.

7. Diet

The need for adequate nutrition during therapy may require frequent food and supplements with a high sugar content. Once the patient is starting to recover, a less cariogenic diet should be resumed.

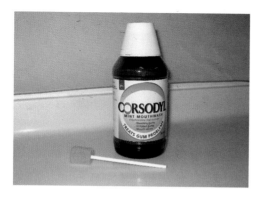

Fig 8-5 Oral hygiene aids during radiotherapy.

Oral Review

As soon as they are well enough, patients should be seen for review by the dental practitioner responsible for their care, to address any problems and to reassess how they are managing their oral care.

Periodontal disease may be exacerbated by oral flora changes, reduced saliva, immunosuppression and pain from mucositis. Once the mucositis lessens, oral hygiene becomes easier and emphasis can be placed on the prevention of dental disease. Those patients who have had extensive surgery to the tongue or floor of the mouth, or who have post-surgical anaesthesia can have difficulty using a toothbrush and invariably need the advice and support of a dental hygienist.

Reduced salivary flow, changes in the oral flora and dietary changes (including build-up foods and frequent drinks to alleviate dry mouth) contribute to increased caries incidence following radiotherapy. "Radiation caries" describes the typical pattern of caries distribution seen in post-radiotherapy patients where the incisal edges of anterior teeth and cusp tips of posterior teeth are affected (Figs 8-6 and 8-7). There may also be root surface caries. A fluoride regime using a daily 0.05% alcohol-free fluoride mouthwash or fluoride gel 1000 ppm in applicator trays for 10 minutes daily should be started to prevent caries (Fig 8-8). Use of high-fluoride toothpaste can also be helpful.

Oral Rehabilitation

Dental treatment may be carried out provided the patient is well and the mouth is not too sore. Treatment may be difficult if there is trismus and,

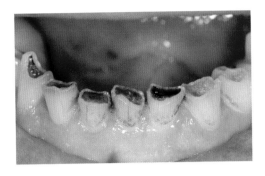

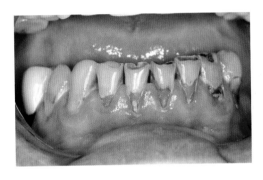

Figs 8-6 and **8-7** Radiation caries.

during treatment, patients may require frequent sips of water and Vaseline for their dry lips. Trismus can also make insertion of dentures and impression taking difficult or sometimes impossible, therefore other options such as resin–retained adhesive bridges and acceptance of the shortened dental arch should be considered. The specialist restorative dentist on the oncol-

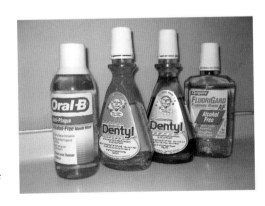

Fig 8-8 Fluoride rinses suitable for daily use after radiotherapy.

ogy team will see patients who have obturators or who require dentures constructed over grafts. Increasingly, the strategic placement of implants is used to aid the retention of prostheses and improve quality of life. However, implants placed in irradiated bone do have a higher than normal failure rate and carry a potential risk of osteoradionecrosis.

Maintenance

Each patient requires a tailored oral health maintenance programme. The dentist on the multidisciplinary oncology team should arrange this with the patient's general dental practitioner. The maintenance programme ensures the mouth is kept healthy and provides regular care and psychological support. It includes:

- regular reviews, at least three-monthly in the first year
- reinforcement of oral hygiene and dietary advice, including use of fluoride supplements and saliva substitutes
- early detection and treatment of caries and periodontal problems, thus avoiding extractions
- denture adjustment/replacement to avoid tissue trauma
- monitoring for recurrent or second primary cancers
- appropriate liaison with the restorative specialist.

Osteoradionecrosis

Radiotherapy causes a reduction in bone vascularity and osteocytes, leading to an increased risk of osteoradionecrosis. This is a serious infection characterised by erythema, swelling, discharge, pain and exposed bone of over three months duration (Fig 8-9). It occurs mainly in patients who received a dose of > 60 Gy, but the susceptibility is always there and increases with time as vascularity diminishes. Osteoradionecrosis is more common in the posterior part of the mandible where the bone is less vascularised, and can result from an extraction, periodontal disease, a dental abscess, a biopsy and even ulceration from a poorly-fitting denture. Its incidence after extractions is around 6%. Any suspected cases should be urgently referred for treatment which can be prolonged and complex, involving antibiotic therapy, bone resection, and in some cases hyperbaric oxygen and ultrasound.

Post-radiotherapy Extraction of Teeth

Extractions following radiotherapy should be avoided, if at all possible, because of the risk of osteoradionecrosis. Careful preradiotherapy assessment

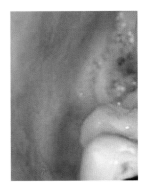

Fig 8-9 Osteoradionecrosis in the retromolar area of the mandible.

and extractions, followed by a preventive programme, and early diagnosis and treatment of disease should make post-radiotherapy extractions a rarity. However, sometimes they will be necessary. Extractions in a field that received > 60 Gy are at significant risk, but a safety margin should be allowed. It is prudent to take precautions for teeth that have been exposed to > 40 Gy. If the total dose or exact field is unknown, or the patient had treatment on an earlier machine where there was more scatter than the present mega-voltage machines, precautions should be taken.

Where possible, post-radiotherapy extractions should be undertaken in a specialist centre. Whilst there are differing views about the antibiotic regime for extractions, the following is a reasonable extraction protocol:

- A suitable antibiotic regime is 3 g amoxicillin orally one hour preoperatively followed by 500 mg amoxicillin tds for 14 days or, if allergic to penicillin, 600 mg clindamycin preoperatively and 200 mg metronidazole tds for 14 days.
- Preoperative oral rinse of 0.2% chlorhexidine mouthwash.
- Extractions carried out with minimal trauma.
- Simple extractions do not require additional intervention, but if the defect is large or bone removal necessary, bone edges should be smoothed and primary tissue closure achieved and sutured in place.
- Normal post-operative instructions should be given and followed.
- Additionally, patients should be told not to smoke, as it increases the risk of osteoradionecrosis.
- Review the patient and if healing is poor, with no granulation tissue covering the bone or an empty socket, further antibiotics should be given – 500 mg amoxicillin tds plus 250 mg tetracycline four times a day for four weeks.

- The socket should continue to be monitored until there is healing. If healing is slow, a dry socket paste may be placed as an antiseptic barrier.

Conclusions

- Cancer of the head and neck region involving surgery or radiotherapy requires a well-planned and coordinated preventive regime and treatment to reduce complications.
- A multidisciplinary team including a restorative dentist and dental hygienist should be in place at head and neck cancer centres to coordinate dental treatment.
- Most of the dental treatment, ongoing maintenance and rehabilitation required by oral cancer patients can be carried out in primary dental care services.

Further Reading

NICE: Improving Outcomes in Head and Neck Cancers. November 2004. www.nice.org.uk

Royal College of Surgeons of England. 1999. The Oral Management of Oncology Patients Requiring Radiotherapy: Chemotherapy: Bone Marrow Transplantation www.rcseng.ac.uk

Useful Web Sites

www.cancerresearchuk.org

www.cancerbacup.org.uk

Chapter 9
Management of Patients With Bleeding Disorders

Aim

The aim of this chapter is to describe the impact of bleeding disorders on the delivery of dental care.

Outcome

After reading this chapter you will have an understanding of how to manage the dental care of patients with bleeding disorders.

Introduction

The most common cause of excessive bleeding is idiopathic, but it can also be caused by:

- anticoagulants
- platelet disorders
- coagulation defects
- rare bleeding disorders.

At some stage every clinician will encounter a patient who complains of excessive bleeding following certain procedures such as dental extractions. The most likely causes are a local problem, or the patient is on anticoagulant medication. However, post-operative bleeding may be one of the first signs of an underlying bleeding disorder, and a small number of patients may require referral for further investigation.

Haemostasis

Haemostasis depends on interactions between the vessel wall, platelets and the clotting pathway. Once a vessel sustains an injury there is an immediate reflex vasoconstriction resulting in a reduced blood flow to the injured area. Damage to the endothelium also activates platelets and the clotting pathway. Activated platelets release agents which act as vasoconstrictors and adhere to collagen in the vessel wall, via specific receptors. The activated platelets spread along the vessel wall to form a subendothelium and the platelet membrane helps to provide a surface for the interaction of coagulation factors so that thrombin encourages platelet fusion. Coagulation is initiated by tissue factor in response to the injury and involves a series of enzymatic reactions (through the intrinsic and extrinsic pathways) leading to the activation of prothrombin and the conversion of soluble plasma fibrinogen to a stable fibrin clot, which is the end point of the clotting cascade.

A bleeding disorder arises if there is a problem in any part of the haemostatic or clotting pathways, and can be acquired or congenital.

Identifying Bleeding Disorders

Ninety per cent of post-operative bleeding is the result of local causes and can be managed using simple haemostatic post-operative measures. A careful medical history helps establish the likelihood of excessive or prolonged bleeding following dental procedures. The factors indicative of a bleeding disorder are outlined in Table 9-1. When a bleeding disorder is confirmed, appropriate measures should be taken to prevent prolonged bleeding as a result of dental procedures. When a bleeding disorder is suspected, referral for investigation prior to undertaking dental treatment likely to cause bleeding is prudent.

1. Anticoagulant Therapy

Anticoagulants provide prophylactic treatment against ischaemic heart disease, myocardial infarction and deep vein thrombosis. Commonly used drugs

Table 9-1 **Indicators of bleeding conditions**

A history of:

Abnormal bruising

Prolonged bleeding from cuts

Nose bleeds, menorrhagia, or haemarthrosis

Haemorrhage following dental extractions, childbirth, or surgery

Previous diagnosis of a bleeding disorder

Family history of a bleeding disorder

Treatment with anticoagulant medication (e.g. aspirin or warfarin)

Liver disease

Table 9-2 **Local measures to achieve haemostasis**

To minimise the risk of post-operative bleeding:
- Carry out all surgery with minimal trauma
- Use a local anaesthetic with a vasoconstrictor
- Use haemostatic agents in sockets (e.g. Surgicell)
- Suture sockets to stabilise gum flaps and avoid clot disturbance
- Use resorbable sutures (e.g. Vicryl)
- Give appropriate post-operative instructions

target platelets (e.g. aspirin), or the clotting pathway (e.g. warfarin). Significant numbers of people are on prescribed anticoagulants and this number is increasing.

a. Anti-platelet therapy
Commonly used drugs include aspirin, or dypiridamol. Many people take aspirin (75 mg daily) to guard against ischaemic heart disease and deep vein thrombosis. This regime does not pose a significant bleeding risk to dental procedures. However, when used in combination, anti-platelet medications have a synergistic effect and impair platelet function for the platelet's lifetime (half-life of 8–12 days).

Management for dental procedures: Current advice from the UK Medicines Information (UKMI) service is that anti-platelet medications (including aspirin in combination with clopidogrel) do not have to be stopped or altered before primary care dental surgical procedures. Locally applied measures are usually adequate to achieve haemostasis (Table 9-2).

b. Coumarin therapy
Warfarin (a vitamin K antagonist) is the most commonly prescribed coumarin, and is used as prophylaxis or treatment in deep vein thrombosis, patients with prosthetic heart valves and people with atrial fibrillation. Warfarin prolongs both the prothrombin time and the activated partial thromboplastin time. Its effects are monitored using the International Normalised Ratio (INR). The usual INR therapeutic range for deep vein thrombosis is 2–3, and up to 4.5 for patients with prosthetic heart valves (Fig 9-1). Whilst there is no such thing as a "safe" INR, generally speaking, the higher the INR the greater the risk of prolonged bleeding.

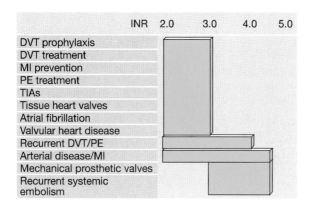

Fig 9-1 Normal therapeutic INR levels.

(DVT = deep vein thrombosis; MI = myocardial infarction; PE = pulmonary embolism; TIAs = transient ischaemic attacks)

Management for dental procedures: Current UKMI advice is that:
- Warfarin does not need to be stopped before dental surgical procedures.
- The risk of thromboembolism after withdrawal of warfarin therapy outweighs the risk of oral bleeding.
- Patients requiring dental surgical procedures in primary care and who have an INR below 4.0 should continue warfarin therapy without dose adjustment.
- Medication should only be stopped or changed under supervision by the anticoagulant clinic.
- Patients on warfarin might bleed more than normal but bleeding is easily treated with local measures.

The administration of inferior dental blocks is considered safe provided the INR is within therapeutic levels. Simple extractions can be carried out using local post-operative haemostatic measures in a general practice setting. People requiring complex/multiple extractions, with a poorly controlled INR, or an INR > 4, should be seen in hospital. It is considered safe to scale a patient on anticoagulants provided the INR is < 4. Even with this knowledge, it is sensible to scale around one or two teeth and observe how long haemostasis takes before proceeding further. Tranexamic mouthwash can be useful for arresting gingival haemorrhage, although its routine use is not recommended as it is expensive and difficult to obtain.

Monitoring the INR: Patients normally carry a record card of their INR readings, from which you can ascertain the average INR and the stability of its control. Erratic differences between INR readings suggest it is poorly controlled. The INR must be checked within the 24-hour period prior to treatment, and ideally on the day of the procedure. This can be reliably done using a self-testing machine such as the Coagucheck monitor (Fig 9-2). This gives an INR value straight away whilst the patient is in the surgery and avoids the need to send the patient to their doctor or Haematology clinic.

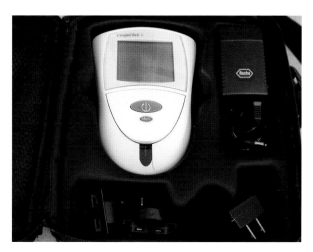

Fig 9-2 Coagucheck monitor.

Warfarin and other drugs: Most of the drugs that interact with warfarin enhance its effect, leading to an elevated INR and risk of spontaneous bleeding. All antibiotics affect the INR value to some extent, although single-dose amoxicillin for antibiotic cover for patients with prosthetic heart valves has little effect. Metronidazole potentiates the effect of warfarin by increasing free warfarin and raising the INR. It should be avoided if possible. If it is necessary to prescribe antibiotics it is important to consult the haematologist/anticoagulation clinic so that the INR value can be monitored during antibiotic therapy. Antifungal agents (such as fluconazole, miconazole, and ketoconazole) potentiate the effect of warfarin severalfold, even after topical use, and must be avoided. It is prudent to refer to the latest Dental Practitioners' Formulary for possible interactions before prescribing for patients taking warfarin.

2. Platelet Disorders
Platelet function can be impaired due to a decrease in number (thrombocytopenia), an increase in number (thrombocytosis), a qualitative disorder or a disturbance in platelet function.

a. Thrombocytopenia
Thrombocytopenia exists when the platelet count falls below $100 \times 10^9/l$. Drugs, bone marrow invasion, autoimmune diseases, and rare platelet disorders can lead to thrombocytopenia. Clinical signs include petechiae, purpura, ecchymoses, nose bleeds, bleeding from the gingivae and postoperative bleeding. Spontaneous bleeding can occur if platelet levels fall below $30 \times 10^9/l$. Major haemorrhage is rare.

Management for dental procedures: A current platelet count is needed to decide where, and how, patients are managed (Table 9-3). A detailed medical history and dental examination are essential. The patient's haematologist should be consulted to discuss:
- the severity of the condition
- the dental treatment planned and the severity of the bleeding risk
- the patient's response to previous dental treatment, surgery and trauma
- the patient's response to systemic therapy to replace platelets.

In patients with idiopathic thrombocytopenia, the bleeding is often effectively controlled with corticosteroids. However, platelet infusions can be indicated in patients with low platelet levels.

b. HIV infection
Purpura are commonly seen in patients with HIV infection. The cause is usually autoimmune, but there may be a platelet defect because of the infection or as a side-effect of the antiviral treatment. Bone marrow disease can also be a contributing factor.

3. Congenital Clotting Disorders
The most common disorders are:
- Haemophilia A
- Haemophilia B (Christmas disease), and
- Von Willebrand's disease.

The precautions that need to be taken during invasive dental procedures likely to cause haemorrhage (such as deep scaling, extractions or administration of inferior dental nerve block injection) depend on the severity of the bleeding disorder. Oral healthcare for people with inherited bleeding disorders should focus on prevention of disease (including dietary advice, use of fluorides, and, in children, fissure sealants), maintaining good oral hygiene and regular review for early detection and treatment of developing disease. For adolescents, planning the management of orthodontic problems is important.

Table 9-3 **Platelet counts and dental management**

Platelet count	Tendency to bleed	Dental management
> 100 x 10^9/L	None	Routine management.
50–100 x 10^9/L	Mild post-operative bleeding	Local measures for a single extraction. Consult regarding platelet cover for multiple extractions. Count of 75 x 10^9/l is desirable for major oral surgery.
< 50 x 100^9/L	Prolonged bleeding post-operatively	May require platelet cover. Refer to a hospital. Avoid ID blocks due to risk of haematoma.
25–50 x 10^9/L	Moderate to severe bleeding post-operatively	Requires platelet cover. Refer to hospital. Avoid ID blocks due to risk of haematoma.
< 25 x 10^9/L	Severe to life-threatening bleeding post-operatively	Requires platelet cover. Refer to hospital. Avoid ID blocks due to risk of haematoma. Avoid surgery.

a. Haemophilia A (Factor VIII deficiency)
This is the most commonly inherited bleeding disorder, although around one third of cases have no family history. It has a prevalence of 1 per 10,000 of the population. It is inherited as a sex-linked recessive trait and therefore affects males. Although females are carriers of the condition, this does not necessarily exclude them from exhibiting symptoms of haemophilia.

Factor VIII is a glycoprotein consisting of:
- Factor VIIIC which participates in the clotting cascade
- Factor VIIIR:Ag – Von Willebrand's Factor which binds to platelets and is the carrier for Factor VIIIC, and
- Factor VIIIR:CO – a cofactor which supports platelet aggregation.

In Haemophilia A only Factor VIIIC is reduced. The severity of haemophilia is related to the Factor VIIIC activity measured by the Factor VIII plasma level (Table 9-4). People with levels over 25% lead relatively normal lives.

Haemophilia can become apparent when there is bleeding into muscles or joints. If haemarthrosis is recurrent, deformity and, in extreme cases, joint replacement can result. More seriously, bleeding into the cranium after a mild head injury can lead to fatal complications. In some cases, post-extraction bleeding can lead to the diagnosis of haemophilia. Unfortunately bleeding into the larynx or the pharynx, due to persistent oozing sometime after the dental work has been completed, can obstruct the airway with fatal consequences. The oozing is delayed due to the initial vascular and platelet response of the haemostatic process.

Table 9-4 **Factor VIII levels and effects**

% Factor VIII activity	Effects
> 25%	Relatively normal life
	Major trauma or surgery can result in prolonged bleeding
5–20%	Mild disease
	Minor trauma leads to persistent bleeding
1–5%	Moderate disease
	Post-traumatic bleeding
< 1%	Severe disease
	Spontaneous bleeding
	Joint deformity if not adequately treated

Management for dental procedures: The concern related to dental procedures is the ability to control post-operative bleeding as this cannot be controlled by local measures alone. The severity of bleeding depends on the level of Factor VIIIC activity and the severity of trauma. Whilst people with mild haemophilia may not bleed excessively following a simple dental extraction, most people with haemophilia will bleed excessively following more traumatic surgery such as surgical third molar removal. Patient management requires liaison with the Haemophilia Centre that helps the patient manage their condition.

The coagulant cover required prior to dental treatment consists of raising the existing Factor VIII levels to normal to achieve adequate haemostasis. Provided this is achieved, most people can receive routine dental treatment (including simple extractions) in the primary dental care setting.

Normal Factor VIII levels can be achieved using:
- Desmopressin (DDAVP®), a synthetic hormone, that induces the release of Factor VIIIC, Von Willebrand's Factor and tissue plasminogen activator from vascular endothelium. It can be given as an intravenous infusion or an intranasal spray.
- Fibrinolytic agents such as tranexamic acid (Cyklokapron) in a dose of 1 g orally four times daily. Tranexamic acid can also be used topically as a mouthwash, 10 ml of a 4.8% solution, for 2 minutes, four times daily for up to 7 days. It can be prescribed for hospital use but is not readily available in the community.
- Replacement Factor VIII which is now genetically engineered rather than harvested from donors.

Most people with mild or moderate haemophilia are used to managing their own coagulant cover and will do so before dental treatment. Additionally, most severely affected patients self-administer Factor VIII at home three times weekly to prevent permanent joint damage. They manage their own cover and can do so for dental treatment in the primary care setting. Caution should still be exercised and dental treatment should be as atraumatic as possible. For example, taking care in placing rubber dam clamps and matrix bands, avoidance of suction injuries, and use of periodontal membrane analgesia.

For minor surgery, such as dental extractions, a Factor VIII level between 50 and 75% is required. Most patients can be managed post-operatively with tranexamic acid and local measures. If local bleeding persists post-operatively, Factor VIII must be given to manage the bleeding problem. If the patient is having a general anaesthetic they must be given replacement Factor VIII to be adequately prepared for endotracheal intubation which is likely to cause bleeding from nasal trauma. Any major surgery should be undertaken by a specialist in a hospital setting in liaison with the patient's medical consultant.

Other Barriers/Challenges

There are a number of other issues that need to be considered in providing oral healthcare for this group:

i. Infection with Blood-borne Viruses – some people contracted blood-borne infections as a result of unscreened, contaminated blood products used until the mid-1980s. For example, in the UK, around 4800 people were infected with hepatitis C and around 1300 with HIV. People who were infected have reported their viral status as a barrier to receiving routine care in general dental practice.

ii. Inhibitors to Factor VIII – between 15 and 25% of patients develop inhibitors to Factor VIII, therefore reducing its activity. This can make their condition more difficult to control. In patients with low titres of inhibitors Factor VIII administration can still be effective. In patients with a high titre of inhibitors, dental treatment likely to cause haemorrhage needs to be carefully planned with the Haemophilia Consultant. Treatment episodes should be planned to minimise the number of times cover needs to be given.

iii. Analgesia – patients must always be advised against taking aspirin or non-steroidal anti-inflammatory drugs as their anti-platelet effect can encourage bleeding. Paracetamol and codeine are safer alternatives for post-operative pain relief.

iv. Anxiety – adults with inherited bleeding disorders have four main sources of anxiety related to dental treatment that need to be addressed. They are:
• the dentist's understanding of their condition and its management
• the dentist's anxiety in providing their dental treatment
• disclosing medical history details that carry a degree of stigma such as positive hepatitis or HIV status, and
• anxiety related to the potential pain/unpleasantness of operative dentistry.

New patients often have poor oral health as a result of a combination of these factors and may require complex dental treatment such as dental extractions or advanced restorative work by the time they present to a dentist who can/will treat them.

v. Mobility Problems – haemarthrosis and resultant joint deformities/replacements can lead to access and mobility problems in gaining access to dental care (see Chapter 2).

b. Haemophilia B (Christmas Disease)
This is a Factor IX deficiency. It has a similar pattern of inheritance, and is clinically identical to Haemophilia A, but is less common.

Management for dental procedures: Coagulant cover is with freeze-dried, genetically modified Factor IX. Oral healthcare considerations are the same as for people with Haemophilia B, with the focus on prevention.

c. Von Willebrand's Disease
This is the most common inherited bleeding disorder and affects about 1% of the population. It has a dominant inheritance pattern and both sexes are affected equally. Von Willebrand's Factor is a carrier protein for Factor VIII. It increases the half-life of Factor VIII and aids platelet adhesion to damaged endothelium. Thus, it is a disorder of platelet adhesion associated with low Von Willebrand's Factor and low Factor VIII activity. If the disorder is mild, it may not be detected until later in life and can go undiagnosed until there is an episode of prolonged bleeding related to an event such as childbirth or a dental extraction.

Management for dental procedures: There are fewer complications than in haemophilia but a greater tendency to more troublesome post-operative bleeding. Cover is provided with Factor VIII concentrate or with DDAVP. Oral healthcare considerations are the same as for people with haemophilia, with the focus on prevention.

4. Vitamin K Deficiency and Malabsorption
Vitamin K is a fat soluble vitamin used to synthesise Factors II, VII, X and XI in the liver, thus, vitamin K deficiency results in prolonged bleeding. People at risk of vitamin K deficiency include those:
- taking aspirin and warfarin
- with insufficient absorption due to obstructive jaundice or malabsorption
- with severe liver disease due to alcoholism, hepatitis or liver cancer.

Its management depends on the cause of the deficiency.

Conclusions
- Most people with acquired or inherited bleeding disorders can be treated in the primary dental care setting.

- Dental care should focus on prevention and routine review.
- Procedures likely to cause haemorrhage should be carefully planned in order to minimise the number of times anticoagulant therapy need be disrupted or coagulant cover need be given.

Further Reading

Fiske J, Pitt Ford HE, Savidge GF, Smith MP. The expressed dental needs of patients attending a Haemophilia Reference Centre. J Disability and Oral Health 2000;1:20-25.

Fiske J, McGeoch RJ, Savidge GF, Smith MP. The treatment needs of adults with bleeding disorders. J Disability and Oral Health 2002;3:59-61.

Lee APH, Boyle CA, Savidge GF, Fiske J. Effectiveness in controlling haemorrhage after dental scaling in people with Haemophilia by using Tranexamic acid mouthwash. Br Dent J 2005;198:33-38.

Chapter 10
Managing Pronounced Gag Reflexes

Aim

The aim of this chapter is to describe the aetiologies and classification of gagging and to provide some practical and useful methods of providing oral healthcare for people with pronounced gag reflexes.

Outcome

By the end of the chapter you should be able to assess the factors that may contribute to patients' gagging problems and produce flexible management strategies for this group of patients.

Introduction

Gagging is a normal reflex. It is designed to be protective and prevent entry of unwanted material into the oropharynx, upper airway and gastrointestinal tract. A pronounced gag reflex can severely affect a patient's ability to accept oral healthcare and your ability to provide it. In its severest form it can compromise all areas of dentistry, from simple diagnostic procedures to any form of active treatment. It will influence treatment planning decisions and may be a major contributing factor to avoidance of treatment by patients. Many techniques have been described to overcome gagging reflexes. Whilst there are no data to demonstrate the prevalence of gagging in the general population, you will undoubtedly see patients with such problems and need knowledge of a variety of management strategies to aid the delivery of oral healthcare.

What is Gagging?

The terms gagging and retching are often used synonymously, but have been interpreted differently in the literature, with gagging considered as "a protective reflex to prevent unwanted entry to the mouth and oropharynx", and retching considered as "the process of attempting to eliminate noxious substances from the upper gastrointestinal tract". Most definitions do not include the psychological and higher cranial centre involvement in gagging even though many dental research articles focus on this aspect. For the purposes of this book, the following practical definition of gagging has been adopted: gagging is a stimulated, protective, reflex response to prevent material from entering the mouth or oropharynx. Gagging stimuli may be physical, auditory, visual, olfactory or psychologically mediated and the muscular contractions provoked may result in vomiting.

During the reflex, the trigeminal, glossopharyngeal and vagus nerves transmit sensory impulses from receptors around the tongue, mouth and oropharynx to the brain. These stimuli may be modulated by impulses received from the olfactory, optic and auditory nerves and by the higher centres (through learned behaviours, emotions and memory). The sensory impulses are mediated in the brain within a number of cranial centres. The vomiting centre lies in the medulla oblongata and is closely linked to the vasomotor, respiratory, salivary and vestibular centres. The efferent control of gagging and retching is relayed from the brain to the muscles of the oropharynx, tongue and upper gastrointestinal tract through the trigeminal, facial, vagus and hypoglossal nerves (and some spinal sympathetic nerves) to the muscles of the stomach and diaphragm.

The fact that gagging can be affected by non-physical stimuli such as sight, hearing and smell reinforces the fact that it is not just a simple reflex but is influenced by higher-centre control. This, in turn, can be subject to abnormal, learned processes or reactions to stressful and distressing events in the past. Some patients can link the onset of their gagging directly to a distressing episode.

The Classification of Gagging

Gagging has been described as simply "psychogenic" or "somatogenic" in origin where the reflex originates either from a psychological or physical stimulus.

- Psychogenic gagging can be induced without direct physical contact and, in its most severe form, just the thought of dental intervention may be sufficient to induce gagging.
- Somatogenic gagging results from direct contact with a specific trigger area. Areas such as lateral borders of the tongue, or certain parts of the palate, are common sites.

These classifications are a little simplistic as most gagging reflexes seen clinically are not wholly one or the other but have components of both psychogenic and somatogenic origin.

The Aetiology of Gagging

There is probably a multifactorial cause for gagging. If it were purely somatically induced then gagging induced by dental instruments would be reproduced by other objects, such as a fork during eating. Most patients who gag at the dentist can eat and place other objects in their own mouths with little or no effect, although some report gagging during tooth brushing. Aetiological factors such as abnormal regional anatomy, oral (hyper) sensitivity and various medical conditions have been postulated but there is little evidence to support these observations. It may be that the primary aetiology is psychogenic and other factors contribute to the severity.

Contributing Factors

A number of influencing or contributing factors have been described and are listed in Table 10-1 in four main categories: Anatomical, Medical, Psychological and Iatrogenic. Many of these factors are included based on clinical observations, and statistical association has not been possible due to the subjective nature of the data and limited sample sizes. Consequently these associations must be viewed with caution but not dismissed outright as statistical "proof" may never be possible.

Assessment of the Nature and Severity of the Gagging Problem

Careful and considerate assessment, starting with a good history, will build rapport and understanding between you and the patient with a gagging problem. Patient confidence is promoted when a patient feels you are taking their problem seriously. They may find their gagging problem embarrassing and difficult to discuss. Open questioning will help the patient to explain the problem in their own terms, provide an indication of any areas of previous treatment success, and help you to understand the most significant issues. It also allows a pre-examination estimation of gagging severity which can be recorded using the index shown in Table 10-2. You need to be aware of the possible limits to future examination and treatment. For example, the treatment possibilities of someone with a history of mild gagging during impression taking will be totally different from someone that gags when a mirror is simply placed behind the upper incisor teeth.

Simple, open questions such as "describe to me the problems you have had with gagging during dental treatment" can be enough to allow you to ask more specific questions later. Some patients may be able to specify exactly

Table 10-1 **Factors contributing to the aetiology of gagging**

Category of contributing factors	Factors
Anatomical	1. Resorption of the maxillary alveolar bone 2. Posterior point and angle of the soft palate 3. Posterior point of the tongue 4. Palatopharyngeal and linguopharyngeal airway 5. Anterior position of the hyoid and the nasopharyngeal isthmus
Medical	1. Nasal obstruction, chronic catarrh, congestion, sinusitis and post-nasal drip 2. Heavy smoking and alcoholism 3. Peptic ulceration and diaphragmatic hernia 4. Pancreatic and glossopharyngeal neoplasms 5. Gilles de Tourette syndrome and other neuropsychiatric and movement disorders 6. Motor neurone disease
Psychological	1. Stress, apprehension, anxiety, fear and phobia 2. Visual, olfactory and audible sounds of dentistry 3. Negative past experiences (real or imagined) 4. Hyperventilation 5. Neuroticism and eating disorders

Iatrogenic	1. Manipulation of the oral tissues with fingers, instruments, equipment, air or water spray
	2. Poor technique by dental staff during treatment, suction or radiography
	3. Denture design characteristics including:
	  – Inadequate posterior palatal and peripheral seal
	  – Restricted tongue space
	  – Over-extension of the posterior palatal border
	  – Excessive thickness of the posterior palatal border
	  – Loss of normal palatal contour
	  – Generalised poor retention or stability for any reason
	  – Incorrect occlusal planes
	  – Reduced or excessive freeway space
	  – Incorrect denture tooth positions

the causes and trigger factors for their gagging problems (for example, a specific event or a particular dental procedure), whilst others will not be able to.

The classification of somatogenic or psychogenic gagging can help the clinician consider the possible strategies required to deal with the problem. Simple somatogenic gagging may be mapped using a ball-ended burnisher and treatment will need simply to avoid these areas – not always as easy as it sounds! Psychogenic gagging problems may require therapeutic assessment and treatment warranting referral to the appropriate counselling services. Most gagging problems appear multifactorial and the clinician may need to use a selection of management techniques to achieve success. The severity of a gagging reflex can simply be described as mild, moderate or severe. The severity index in Table 10-2 describes gagging severity in terms of its induction and the prevention methods that may be necessary to allow treatment. It can be used as an initial baseline assessment against which you can measure the success of any management strategies later.

Clinical Examination

Traffic lights: Some patients require gagging control methods even for a simple visual clinical examination. It is useful to have a signalling system organised that allows the patient control during the examination. The "Traffic Light" hand signalling system is very useful (Figs 10-1a–c). The three positions (green, amber and red) inform you whether you should continue (green), take care (amber) or stop (red) during the examination/treatment episode. Just before the gagging point is reached the patient changes the hand from horizontal to a vertical stop signal. It must be explained to the patient that the red "stop" signal is given to show that the patient wants the treatment to stop before gagging commences. Continuing until the patient gags will just negatively reinforce the reflex and reduce the patient's confidence in you.

Avoidance: With psychogenic gagging certain sounds, sights, smells, materials or instruments may need to be avoided, hidden or disguised. Personal stereos and perfumes can be used by patients to mask the sounds of drills, suction and the smell of some dental materials. Diagnostic radiography can be very difficult and may need specific measures to achieve success. Often extra oral radiography is all that can be performed. The DPT radiograph shown in Fig 10-2, illustrates acupuncture needles in place (visible at the edges of the film) to control a severe gagging reflex (GSI IV) in a patient that gagged even when the anterior bite block was placed between the front teeth.

119

Table 10-2 **Gagging Severity Index (GSI)**

Severity grading	Description
Grade I Normal gagging reflex	**Very occasional gagging** Occurs during high-risk dental procedures such as maxillary impression taking or restoration to the distal, palatal or lingual surfaces of molar teeth. This is basically a "normal" gag reflex under difficult treatment circumstances. *Generally controlled by the patient*
Grade II Mild gagging	**Occasional gagging** Occurs occasionally during routine dental procedures such as fillings, scaling and impressions. *Control can usually be regained by the patient*, but may need assistance and reassurance from members of the dental team, and treatment continued. Generally, no special measures are needed to facilitate routine treatment but may be required for more difficult procedures
Grade III Moderate gagging	**Regular gagging** Occurs routinely during normal dental procedures. This may include simple physical examination of high-risk areas, such as the lingual aspect of lower molars. Recommencement may be difficult. The gag reflex may influence treatment planning and may limit treatment options. Gagging prevention measures are usually required. *Once instigated, the patient has difficulty regaining control* without cessation of the procedure
Grade IV Severe gagging	**Gagging occurs with all forms of dental treatment including simple visual examination** Routine treatment is impossible without some form of special measure to attempt to control the gag reflex. Treatment options may be limited and the gagging problem will be a major factor in treatment planning. *The patient cannot control it*
Grade V Very severe gagging	**Gagging occurs easily and may not necessarily require physical intervention to trigger the reflex** It will be one of the prime factors when planning treatment. Treatment options may be severely limited. Dental treatment will be impossible to carry out without specific, special treatment for control of the gagging problem. *The patient's behaviour and dental attendance may be governed by the gagging problem*

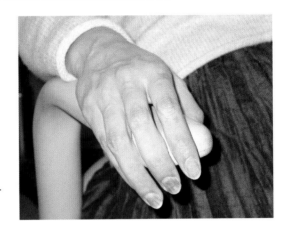

Fig 10-1a Traffic light position – green for continue.

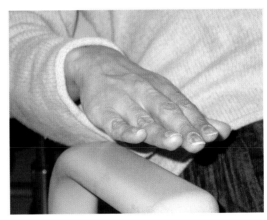

Fig 10-1b Traffic light position – amber for take care.

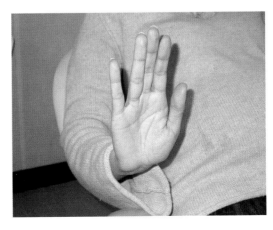

Fig 10-1c Traffic light position – red for stop.

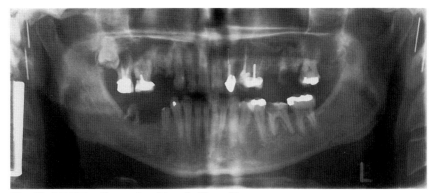

Fig 10-2 DPT radiograph-taking facilitated by ear acupuncture.

Initial Treatment

Once the oral assessment is completed you must link the severity of the gagging reflex with the complexity of the treatment required to formulate a treatment plan. For example, the need for a molar endodontic treatment on a person with a mild gagging problem (GSI grade II) may be as difficult as lower anterior teeth scaling in someone with a severe reflex (GSI grade IV). You need to make the patient understand the scope of possible treatment to avoid false hopes and disappointments when things do not go as the patient (and you) had hoped. In the early stages of treatment the watchwords of "promise nothing" are sensible. Start with simple procedures and slowly build patient confidence. You may need to use multiple and varied gagging control methods depending on the item of treatment. A simple anterior restoration may need a different level of gagging control to one in an upper molar. Remember also that patients have good and bad times/days, and what succeeded at one appointment may not succeed at the next.

Above all be empathetic and understanding. Patients do not want sympathy. They need a clinician who will:
• take their problem seriously
• persevere with them to overcome the problem
• be flexible in approach.

The value of the calm, confident and "in control" approach to confidence building in the gagging patient has been recognised by many researchers. The "relationship" between the dentist and the patient is central to success.

Some researchers found that the highest percentage of gagging occurred with the least experienced operators.

Gagging Reduction Strategies for Examination and Treatment

Gagging reduction strategies fall into the following categories:
1. relaxation, distraction and desensitisation techniques
2. psychological and behavioural therapies
3. use of pharmacological agents
4. complementary therapies
5. miscellaneous useful techniques.

1. Relaxation, Distraction and Desensitisation Techniques
Relaxation: For some patients their gag reflex is exacerbated by stress and anxiety.

- *Passive relaxation* from the creation of a calming surgery environment by avoiding obvious displays of instrumentation and using relaxing images and music in reception areas and surgeries is helpful.
- *Active relaxation* methods are simple and effective. Slow deep breathing exercises act as a relaxant and distraction by focusing the patient's attention away from the dentistry. Some believe breath-holding and hyperventilation to be factors in gagging modulation and breathing control will help this. Hi-tech solutions include the use of audiovisual devices that the patient wears on their head to watch calming (and distracting) images whilst listening to relaxing music in headphones.

Distraction techniques: These work by diverting the patient's attention away from dentistry long enough to perform a particular procedure. The patient is asked to concentrate on a task or thought that completely absorbs the mind. The following list gives examples of distraction methods that have been used successfully:

- Tasks that absorb thought, such as raising one leg and rotating their foot anticlockwise during impressions.
- Asking a patient to carry out a mental exercise or focus their attention on a complex object.
- Use of semi-hypnotic suggestions by asking the patient to focus on and "visit" a favourite relaxing and pleasant place.
- The "temporal tap" technique, in which you gently tap the temporoparietal suture, prior to, and during, dental procedures as a trigger to a verbal suggestion regarding gagging prevention.
- Table salt poured onto the anterior, dorsum of the tongue for five seconds prior to dental procedures such as radiographs or impressions.

- Simple blindfold for the patient whose gagging reflex is induced by the sight of dental equipment and instruments.
- Rinsing the mouth with ice-cold water prior to intraoral radiography.

Desensitisation techniques: These procedures aim to permanently reduce the threshold of gagging and vomiting. Methods that have been used include:
- Asking patients to keep buttons, marbles, or acrylic discs in the mouth for short periods of time and slowly increasing the number, size or length of time. There are potential choking hazards of advocating use of these items. This can be overcome by securing them extra-orally with lengths of dental floss for safety.
- Training plates – sandblasted toothless training base plates can be constructed for denture wearers and soft "blow down" splints or small "orthodontic" plates can be used for dentate patients.
- Acrylic beads added to training plates give a focus for the tongue.
- Other "homework" items include flexible suction tips, radiographic beam aiming devices, occlusal radiographs, impression trays and mouth mirrors (Fig 10-3). The advantage of this technique is that the patient can get used to placing items, such as dental mirrors or impression trays, in their own mouth in the comfort of their own home and in their own time.

2. Psychological and Behavioural Therapies
Psychoanalytical and psychotherapeutic techniques are specialist techniques and not for the dental practitioner. Dentists regularly use simple behavioural techniques such as "ego enhancement" and "confidence building", often in

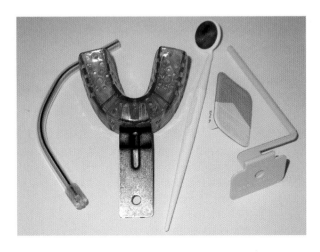

Fig 10-3 "Homework" items used for desensitisation.

conjunction with distraction and relaxation. Simple strategies such as "mock" rehearsals of dental procedures using the "tell–show–do" approach, prior to actual treatment can be helpful. Anxiety reduction techniques, such as biofeedback and visualisation during techniques to alter ingrained behavioural patterns, and behavioural therapy techniques such as reframing and flooding are the realm of the specialist.

3. Pharmacological Agents – Local Anaesthesia, Sedation and General Anaesthesia

Application of local anaesthetic preparations, either by injection or topical application has been used to try to prevent gagging. Infiltration and block local analgesia can be useful if the aetiology is purely somatogenic. In gagging of psychogenic origin anaesthetising the mouth can produce the opposite effect as some patients react to the "swollen" feel of the oral tissues. Topically applied local analgesics are unlikely to work as they diffuse poorly through palatal keratinised mucosa and have a limited working time.

Gagging control has been reported using:
- inhalation sedation with nitrous oxide and oxygen
- intravenous sedation with midazolam
- intravenous sedation with propofol.

Nitrous oxide can give a constant depth of sedation and so can be useful in longer dental procedures. Intravenous techniques produce a more profound gag suppressive effect at the beginning of the sedation but gagging can return as the sedation wears off. General anaesthesia, generally used as a last resort, is the only method of guaranteeing control of gagging.

4. Complementary Therapies

Acupuncture, acupressure, transcutaneous electrical nerve stimulation (TENS) and hypnosis have all been used to help people overcome gagging problems.

Acupuncture and acupressure: These both stimulate specific points on the body. The former utilises fine needles to puncture the skin and the latter uses direct pressure without puncturing the skin. Several reported acupuncture points have been used to control dental gagging and/or nausea. Common points used are the labiomental fold point (CV24, Fig 10-4); PC6 (Xianyun), an antinausea point which lies on the medial side of the forearm; and L4 (Hegu) which lies in the concave area between the first and second metacarpal bones of the hand.

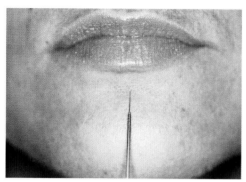

Fig 10-4 Acupuncture needle in CV24 to control gagging.

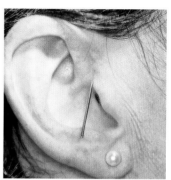

Fig 10-5 Ear acupuncture point used to control gagging.

PC6 is the pressure point utilised by commercially available travel sickness bands. Ear acupuncture points have been used successfully to reduce gagging (Fig 10-5). Acupuncture is a skill requiring training and experience.

Transcutaneous electrical nerve stimulation: TENS has been used for stimulation of the PC6 point to successfully control nausea.

Hypnosis: This has been used as a symptomatic adjunct to dental treatment as well as a treatment for the gag reflex itself. Hypnotherapeutic desensitisation would seem the preferable course of action with the aim of permanent reduction or abolition of the profound gag reflex associated with dental treatment. There appear to be few contraindications to its use but results can be variable. Hypnosis is recognised for treatment of phobias and addictions such as flying and smoking. The subconscious psychogenic component of gagging lends itself to treatment by hypnosis.

5. Other Techniques
There are a number of other simple techniques that can help to prevent stimulation of the gag-reflex:

- Perforated impression trays can be a particular problem for gagging patients and non-perforated special trays should be requested.
- The use of quick-setting impression materials in carefully constructed special trays or sectional impression trays.
- Creating a post-dam in impression compound prior to impression taking prevents excess material escaping from the tray towards the oropharynx.

- Use of rubber dam to prevent:
  – the air or water spray triggering the gag reflex
  – debris falling on the tongue or other sensitive areas
  – the need to use suction at the back of the mouth
  and to provide a psychological "curtain" between the patient and the dental treatment.
- Closed mouth techniques for inferior alveolar block analgesia.

Recording Success

Any reduction in gagging can be assessed using the Gagging Prevention Index (Table 10-3) and compared with the Gagging Severity Index score seen on initial consultation. This will give you and the patient valuable

Table 10-3 **Gagging Prevention Index (GPI)**

Prevention grading	Description
Grade I Gagging reflex obtunded	Treatment and management methods employed at this visit totally obtund the gag reflex. *Proposed treatment was completely successful*
Grade II Partial control	Partial control of the gag reflex. *The proposed treatment was possible but occasional gagging occurred*
Grade III Partial control	Partial control of the gag reflex. Gagging occurred frequently. *The proposed treatment was part completed or alternative treatment involving simpler procedures was carried out*
Grade IV Inadequate control	Inadequate control of the gag reflex. Gagging occurred regularly. *The proposed treatment was not possible; some "treatment" was carried out but only very simple procedures*
Grade V No control	Failure to control the gag reflex. *Gag reflex was so severe that no treatment was possible. Even simple treatment procedures not possible*

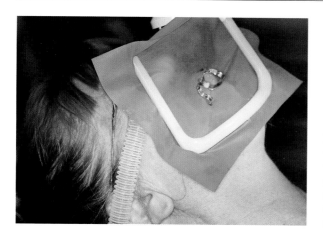

Fig 10-6 A combination of ear acupuncture, nitrous oxide inhalation sedation and rubber dam used to control a severe gag reflex.

objective feedback on the gagging management strategies. It will then allow flexible strategies to be developed to control the reflex for the different items of treatment the patient may need. Often multiple strategies need to be employed during a treatment plan. A patient with a severe gagging reflex (GSI IV) undergoing endodontic treatment using ear acupuncture, nitrous oxide inhalation sedation and rubber dam is shown in Fig 10-6. The gagging reflex was totally obtunded (GPI). This was the first treatment this patient had managed to accept in over 10 years.

Conclusions

- You need to be aware of the aetiological and modulating factors for gagging reflexes.
- Overcoming gagging problems requires the combination of a careful history with individually tailored, flexible treatment planning by a knowledgeable, experienced and empathetic dental team.
- There is no magic bullet, and it may be necessary to try a number of techniques or a combination of techniques to find something that helps.

Further Reading

Bassi GS, Humphris GM, Longman LP. The aetiology and management of gagging: a review of the literature. J Prosthet Dent 2004;91:459-467.

Dickinson CM, Fiske J. A review of gagging problems in dentistry: I. Aetiology and classification. Dent Update 2005;32:26-32.

Dickinson CM, Fiske J. A review of gagging problems in dentistry: 2. Clinical assessment and management. Dent Update 2005;32:74-80.

Chapter 11
Patient Management Through Non-invasive Treatment

Aim

The aim of this chapter is to describe non-invasive operative procedures that can be used as an alternative to conventional techniques such as local anaesthetic injection and the dental drill.

Outcome

After reading this chapter you should be aware of the techniques that are available as an alternative to current conventional invasive restorative techniques and understand when they are useful.

Introduction

Rotary instruments and hand excavators are routinely used to remove caries during operative treatment of cavitated carious lesions in dentine. Unfortunately, these conventional techniques have several drawbacks including bone-conducted vibrations, high-pitched noise of the air-turbine, sensitivity of vital dentine, development of high temperatures at the cutting surface leading to thermal stimulation as well as possible over-preparation of the cavity. Combined, they are responsible for causing discomfort and pain to the patient. Even if the operator tries to minimise these disagreeable aspects of cavity preparation by keeping the bur speed and pressure constant they are not completely eradicated and local anaesthesia is required. Local anaesthetic injections and the use of dental handpieces and burs are well-documented triggers of dental anxiety.

Anxiety is a well-recognised barrier to the receipt of dental care that can lead to avoidance behaviours and, thus, can have a detrimental effect on oral health. Consequently, people with severe dental anxiety are often in pain and require complex treatment by the time they present to the dentist. In some instances anxiety is such that treatment under sedation or general anaesthesia is required (see Chapter 12), but in others the use of non-invasive treatment can be helpful in building trust, rapport and communication. Coping with conventional techniques can also be difficult for other groups of people to deal with and may be part of the reason why people with learning disabilities have more missing than restored teeth compared with the general population. Whilst it is accepted that the preferred dental management of people requiring Special Care Dentistry is the prevention of dental disease (thus removing the need for invasive dental treatment), in reality, this is not always an achievable goal. In circumstances where dental disease already exists and its treatment is required, the goal must be to make the treatment experience as acceptable as possible. This can be achieved with the use of dental techniques that are as non-invasive and as atraumatic as possible.

Alternative Operative Techniques

Techniques that can help overcome the common triggers of dental anxiety include:

1. Atraumatic Restorative Technique (ART)

ART is based on excavating carious cavities using hand instruments only and using adhesive filling material, such as a glass-ionomer cement, for subsequent restoration. This technique was originally developed to bridge the gap in provision of dental treatment in Tanzania, and aimed at treating people living in rural areas in developing countries where installation of appropriate treatment facilities is difficult, as it does not require the use of drills, running water or electricity. In 1994, the regulation and promotion of this technique were fostered by the World Health Organization. The technique has been widely used since then and evaluation of restorations placed using ART shows satisfactory results at six months, one year, and three years. It is a simple, quick and inexpensive technique requiring no special equipment.

Its minimal intervention approach provides an excellent alternative for:
- children who are being introduced to dental treatment
- patients who experience extreme fear or anxiety about dental procedures
- people who require domiciliary care
- people who are unable to tolerate more conventional restorative treatment, such as patients with a learning disability, dementia, etc.
- people who have movement disorders that can make the use of some dental equipment hazardous, such as athetoid cerebral palsy.

2. Air Abrasion

Air abrasion, developed by Robert Black in 1945, was designed to supplement the conventional high-speed air turbine to avoid its unwanted effects of vibrations, pressure, heat production and pulpal reactions. It is a pseudo-mechanical, non-rotary method that uses kinetic energy to cut dental hard tissues and composite or porcelain restorations. Recent advances in dental technology and adhesive materials permitting minimal cavity preparation, improved isolation using the rubber dam technique and high-volume suction apparatus have led to a renewed interest in the air abrasion technique. Air abrasion can abrade carious enamel and sound dentine painlessly by blasting the tooth with high-velocity alumina particles at a pressure between 60 and 120 p.s.i., depending on the diameter of the nozzle tip. The energy is transferred to the tooth surface on impact and, acting as an end cutting instrument, produces a small diameter access cavity. The proteins in the freshly cut vital dentine tubules coagulate as the air stream passes over them, forming a physiological barrier that prevents further pain stimulation of the dentine-pulp complex.

Advantages of air abrasion
- It is an easy, quick and effective technique.
- It can abrade both enamel and sound dentine efficiently.
- Its cutting characteristics can be controlled by changing the type and size of the alumina particles, the velocity of the particles, the air pressure, the distance between the nozzle tip and tooth, and the length of cutting time.
- It generates less heat, vibration, and mechanical stimulation than is felt with the air-turbine despite local anaesthesia.
- It is relatively pain-free, permitting use without local anaesthesia.

Disadvantages of air abrasion
- Lack of tactile feedback, which can lead to over-preparation of the cavity and cutting into healthy tooth tissue.
- Failure to remove clinically soft carious dentine because of its reduced hardness compared with that of the alumina particles.
- The creation of dust which leads to:
  - the risk of particle inhalation (current systems have full US FDA approval for clinical use of 27.5 micron alumina particles)
  - poor visibility during cavity preparation as the mirror surface becomes covered and needs constant cleaning
  - the need to use rubber dam isolation, facemask protection for the dental team and efficient high-volume suction.
- The technique requires a degree of cooperation and is more suitable to people with anxiety than for those with movement disorder or learning disability.

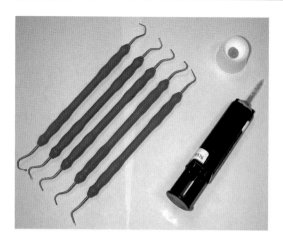

Fig 11-1 Carisolv™ gel delivery system.

Main indications for use
Air abrasion can be used for various clinical purposes provided that direct vision and access with the nozzle are easily achievable. Its uses include:
- Minimal cavity preparations required in preventive resin/sealant restorations, tunnel preparations or class IV and V cavities.
- Labial veneers on anterior teeth can be prepared using this technique and then restored using composite.
- Composite restoration repairs, particularly of large restorations where complete removal would jeopardise the tooth.
- Removal of surface discolouration of existing restorations.
- Removal of extrinsic staining.

Cost
Air abrasion units are relatively expensive. However, cost varies depending on the functions of the unit, such as the inclusion of a built-in high-volume suction unit or pulse system. The powder is relatively inexpensive. The air abrasion method saves time and therefore money, when compared with the conventional method because it can cut tooth tissue rapidly and avoids the necessity of waiting for the local anaesthetic to work.

3. Carisolv™ Gel
Chemomechanical removal of dentine caries was introduced in 1972 in the form of Caridex solution. The technique has been further developed and refined and currently Carisolv™ gel is available to aid carious dentine removal using special non-cutting hand instruments (Fig 11-1). The

aim of chemomechanical caries removal is to chemically disrupt denatured collagen in a demineralised zone and then to remove the unsupported enamel by gentle scraping. This is designed to leave a hard cavity floor with healthy collagen embedded in mineral suitable for etching and bonding procedures.

Carisolv™ gel comes in a single dispenser. It consists of two solutions mixed just before application. They contain a dye, carboxymethylcellulose gel, sodium chloride, purified water and sodium hydroxide with a pH of 11. Approximately 0.5–1 ml of gel is applied to the carious cavity using a non-cutting hand instrument. The gel is left for 60 seconds, or until it turns cloudy, prior to gently but firmly abrading away the softened dentine (Fig 11-2). This stage is repeated until a hard and caries free cavity is achieved. A good clinical indication that the surface is caries free is that the gel remains clear and no longer turns cloudy. Care should be taken not to use a sharp instrument for caries removal to avoid causing pain to the patient.

Advantages of Carisolv™ gel
- It is capable of removing carious dentine as effectively, and more selectively, than is conventional drilling.
- It is safe and has no adverse effects on the pulp or healthy tooth tissue.
- Careful cavity selection and a careful technique make its use pain-free so that in many cases local anaesthesia can be avoided.
- Patient compliance is good compared with that for conventional operative methods such as use of the dental drill or hand excavation to remove caries.

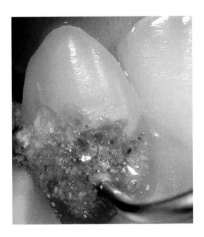

Fig 11-2 Softened dentine being abraded.

Disadvantages of Carisolv™ gel
- It does not penetrate enamel and can only be used on accessible carious dentine.
- The technique has been considered as time-consuming compared with using the air-turbine, but, interestingly, this is not a patient perception.

Main indication for use
Removal of readily accessible caries in situations where patients are:
- anxious
- have difficulty coping or cooperating with the use of the drill
- have movement disorders that make the use of conventional equipment hazardous.

4. Combination of Air Abrasion and Carisolv™ Gel

There is evidence to show that a combination of air abrasion, to gain access through enamel to dentinal caries, and Carisolv™ gel, to remove caries in softened dentine, has resulted in positive patient perception in comparison with the more conventional techniques of using local anaesthesia and the air turbine, in terms of degree of anxiety, taste, numbness and comfort.

5. Oraqix

Oraqix is a subgingival anaesthetic gel that contains 2.5% lidocaine and 2.5% prilocaine, which is indicated for use in scaling. Its unique dispenser allows the liquid gel to be injected into the periodontal pocket, where it gels further, helping it to remain in place. Its speed of onset is 30 seconds and its effect lasts up to 20 minutes. Its use avoids the need to administer local anaesthetic injections for deep scaling. There are, as yet, few studies to demonstrate its performance, however, it seems promising.

6. Ozone

Ozone is a powerful oxidising agent that has a bactericidal effect. It has been used widely for several years to purify water systems, in food preservation, and in equipment sterilisation. Its ability to kill bacteria efficiently has led to the development of its use in dentistry. Delivery systems, such as Healozone, convert oxygen into ozone which is delivered (through a tube and a handpiece with special silicone cups that provide an airtight seal) as a high concentration of gaseous ozone to a precise area on the tooth surface.

Main indications for use
Its main applications are said to be:
- Caries removal from small lesions – the technique involves no injections, no drilling and is pain-free. However, larger lesions require conventional procedures to gain access to the caries.
- Dealing with root caries.
- Fissure-sealing – where ozone can be used to disinfect fissures of the bacteria before they are sealed.
- Reduction of bacterial load – ozone has been shown to significantly reduce the total microbial load within carious lesions as well as reducing isolated strains of *Streptococcus mutans* and *Streptococcus sobrinus* both *in vivo* and *in vitro*. The elimination of these organisms shifts the microbial flora towards less acidogenic micro-organisms, and inhibits recolonisation by cariogenic micro-organisms. Calcium from saliva and toothpastes can then remineralise the damaged tooth surfaces over a period of several weeks.

The evidence to support the efficacy of the use of ozone in restorative dentistry is mixed. When proven, it will have a place in the treatment of older people, as well as anxious children and adults.

Conclusions

- Non-invasive operative techniques can be used to replace more conventional techniques of local anaesthetic injection and the use of the rotary drill.
- These techniques are particularly useful for patients with a low coping threshold and with movement disorders.
- They are also useful where people have a true allergy to more than one local anaesthetic agent, a severe haematological disorder, and medical conditions that can be worsened by anxiety, such as asthma or angina.

Further Reading

Banerjee A, Watson TF. Air abrasion: Its uses and abuses. Dent Update 2002;29:340-346.

Baysan A, Lynch E. Effect of ozone on the oral microbiota and clinical severity of primary root caries. Am Dent J 2004;17:56-60.

Honkala E, Behebehani J, Ibricevic H, Kerosuo E, Al-Jame G. The atraumatic restorative treatment (ART) approach to restoring primary teeth in a standard dental clinic. Int J Paediatr Dent 2003;13:172-179.

Rafique S, Fiske J, Banerjee A. Clinical trial of an air-abrasion/chemomechanical operative procedure for the restorative treatment of dental patients. Caries Res 2003;37:360-364.

Chapter 12

Sedation and General Anaesthesia in Special Care Dentistry

Aim

To describe the different techniques available to manage special care patients who are unable to cope with conventional delivery of dental care and whose treatment needs are beyond those that can be provided by non-invasive techniques.

Outcome

After reading this chapter the practitioner will be aware of the range of available sedation techniques, and the disadvantages/advantages of general anaesthesia (GA), for special care patients.

Introduction

Historically, GA has been used to treat people requiring Special Care Dentistry who had complicated medical histories, or a physical or mental disability making it difficult for them to cooperate with dental care. In addition to their disability, they may also have been anxious. Access to GA has become more difficult subsequent to its restriction to a hospital setting. Aside from access difficulties, GA is not an ideal method of providing dental care as:

- treatment planning can be difficult
- limited time and facilities are available to complete all dental treatment in one session
- a patient who can not be examined preoperatively could be subjected to the inconvenience and risk of GA only to find that no treatment is required
- it is difficult to justify GA to carry out scaling on a regular basis for patients with learning disabilities who are unable to carry out efficient oral hygiene procedures.

Conscious sedation offers an alternative method of behaviour management to GA. Sedative drugs may be administered by a variety of routes each of which have advantages and disadvantages. This chapter describes the use of sedation techniques in providing dental care for adult patients who require special care, and the appropriate use of GA.

Intravenous Sedation (IV)

IV sedation regulations require that dental staff involved in its use have been properly trained and that it is only used in appropriate settings. In the UK the most commonly used IV sedative drug is midazolam. This is a water soluble benzodiazepine with a short half-life that provides:

- rapid onset sedation
- anxiolysis
- anterograde amnesia
- rapid recovery allowing discharge within one or two hours.

It has the disadvantage of requiring venous access, which can be difficult to achieve in uncooperative or anxious patients. Also, midazolam can lead to respiratory depression, particularly in older people or if injected rapidly. For this reason, pulse oximetry is mandatory throughout treatment for all sedation patients. IV sedation can be used for people with learning difficulties if they are able to cooperate with the placement of a cannula. The main challenge, in someone who has little or no verbal communication, is determining the level of sedation and the dental team must rely on observations such as the patient appearing relaxed and accepting dental treatment.

IV sedation can be safer for anxious people with cardiac conditions than local anaesthesia alone, as anxiety is reduced and oxygen saturation can be maintained with supplemental oxygen (two litres per minute via a nasal cannula) throughout treatment. There are also dental advantages in carrying out treatment under sedation in stages rather than in a single GA appointment.

Inhalational Sedation (IS)

IS produces sedation using a mixture of nitrous oxide and oxygen delivered in varying concentrations by a dedicated machine through a nasal mask. Modern machines deliver a minimum of 30% oxygen at all times. Most adults require between 30 and 50% of nitrous oxide for sedation. The technique is operator sensitive as the sedative effect of the nitrous oxide is supplemented by semihypnotic suggestion. IS is an extremely safe technique that can be used to treat adults and children with mild to moderate anxiety, mild to moderate learning disabilities, and medical conditions (such as cardiac defects and angina) that benefit from additional oxygenation. The technique requires patient cooperation and it may not be possible for patients with more severe learning disabilities to understand the suggestions which are important for the success of the technique. It also requires the individual to breathe through their nose only. This is difficult for people with nasal congestion, as is common in Down's syndrome. An advantage of IS is that nitrous oxide has a short half-life and, as a consequence, the technique causes no post-operative drowsiness.

Oral Sedation

Oral sedation offers significant advantages over IV and IS techniques as it avoids the need for intravenous access and requires little patient cooperation. It has the disadvantage of variable absorption due to the effect of anxiety on gut motility and the presence or absence of food in the stomach.

The commonly used oral sedative Temazepam takes two to three hours to reach peak plasma levels. In practice the dentist has to wait at least 40 minutes for effective sedation to be achieved following the administration of 10 to 30 mg of oral Temazepam. This delay can be upsetting for the patient, carers, staff and other patients in the treatment area. However, oral sedation with midazolam provides safe and effective sedation with rapid onset. Peak plasma levels are generally achieved in 30 minutes and dental treatment can usually start 15–20 minutes after administration. If an oral dose does not give adequate sedation for dentistry, sufficient cooperation should be achieved to allow placement of an intravenous line and further increments of intravenous midazolam.

Where midazolam is not yet available as an oral formulation, for example in the UK, an ampoule of 10 mg midazolam in 2 ml may be used. Mixing it with the patient's favourite drink (e.g. tea, squash) and glucose makes it more palatable. The oral use of midazolam is not licensed in some countries. Where this is the case, oral use may still be permitted provided it is considered clinically justifiable and the decision is discussed with the patient, parents and carers. Written consent should be obtained from the patient specifying that midazolam is being used off-licence and the practitioner should be aware of all current information and research on this subject so that actions are evidence-based. Additionally, the supplier (usually the local pharmacy) should be made aware of the proposed unlicensed use of the drug.

Transmucosal Sedation

In transmucosal sedation the sedative agent is administered via the oral, buccal, nasal or rectal mucosa. The last route is not acceptable in the UK, although it is the most commonly used route for sedation in Scandinavia. Intranasal sedation is a useful technique in people with learning disabilities as it requires little cooperation and has a rapid onset. Where midazolam is not licensed for use in this way, it may still be permitted provided it is considered clinically justifiable; the decision is discussed with the patient, parents and carers; written consent is obtained, specifying its use off-licence; the practitioner's actions are evidence-based; and the supplier is aware of the proposed unlicensed use of the drug. The usual dose for an adult is 10 mg, which even in the more concentrated form of 10 mg/2 ml is a large volume to be sprayed up the nostrils. Surprisingly, most patients accept this volume well although trials are being carried out to produce a more concentrated, lower-volume version. Midazolam mixed with glucose syrup for sublingual absorption has been described and has produced promising results in children.

General Anaesthesia

It is estimated that around 20% of people with a severe disability need general anaesthesia to complete dental care. Dental treatment under general anaesthesia should only take place:

- when it is judged to be the most clinically appropriate method of anaesthesia, and
- in a setting that has critical care facilities, usually a hospital.

The types of patients requiring dental care under GA fall into three broad categories:

1. Those who will not allow even an examination when awake and for whom sedation techniques have been unsuccessful. In this group it can be difficult for carers to ascertain whether the person is suffering dental pain and GA may be required for an examination followed by any necessary treatment. This provides particular challenges for the dental team who have to devise a treatment plan in theatre.
2. Those for whom sedation is partially successful and examination and cleaning are possible but operative dentistry is not. This group can have sedation on a regular basis for recalls and oral hygiene measures but require GA for more advanced care.
3. Those for whom sedation allows examination but this reveals either a high volume of treatment need or more difficult dentistry (e.g. surgical removal

of teeth). For these patients the initial examination under sedation allows dental treatment to be planned and discussed before the GA.

Patient Assessment for Anaesthesia

The dentist who is to treat the patient should carry out the dental assessment and ensure that full medical and past anaesthetic histories are available. The amount of information that can be given to the patient and/or carers regarding the treatment planned depends on the ease of dental examination and if preoperative radiographs can be taken. An anaesthetic assessment of fitness will be carried our prior to, or on the day of, the GA. An alternative is for an experienced dentist to make that evaluation discussing cases where there is any uncertainty regarding fitness with the anaesthetist.

Consent should be obtained at the assessment visit. It is important that there is compliance with national guidance on consent. For example, in England, the Department of Health has produced a consent form specifically for adults who are unable to consent to investigation or treatment. It includes details of an assessment of the patient's capacity and best interests and there is space for those close to the patients and for two healthcare professionals to sign the form. In Scotland there are specific procedures and regulations to follow, governed by the Mental Health (Scotland) Act 2003.

It is reasonable that the risks of GA are discussed with the patient and carers. It is not necessary to tell patients that they might die under GA but they can be informed of the current mortality rates. In developed countries this is around one in 400,000, and this risk is considerably less than being seriously injured in a road accident. The limitations in the scope of dental care that can be provided under GA should be discussed and agreement reached that teeth with extensive caries will be extracted and not restored.

The General Anaesthetic Setting

Many general hospitals have purpose-built day-case units with dedicated nursing staff who work to defined protocols. This can sometimes be a difficult environment in which to treat special care patients as they do not always fit day-stay guidelines. For example, it is accepted that day-case surgery should not extend beyond 90 minutes. However, it can be difficult for the dental team to know whether treatment can be completed within that time frame when they are faced with a patient who will not allow a pre-GA oral examination. There are also medical constraints on day-case surgery. For example, patients should not be obese and should have no limiting medical conditions. Sometimes investigations such as a full blood count or chest X-ray would be required before surgery. For some special care patients these investigations are not possible preoperatively. Managing special care patients within a day-case unit requires flexibility on the part of the nursing and medical staff. For example it may be necessary to treat someone with challenging behaviour before other patients arrive; or to treat a medically compromised person as a day stay to avoid hospital admission which would be distressing for them and their families. For the particularly challenging patient, there may be requests to optimise the "dental" GA visit and carry out blood tests, other investigations such as hearing tests, or even other surgery such as chiropody. This requires liaison with other healthcare professionals.

Making the Decision Between Sedation or General Anaesthesia

There are no set rules for deciding whether dental care should be provided under GA or sedation and patients need to be assessed individually. Even if a patient has routinely required GA to facilitate dental treatment in the past, it is worth considering if sedation is a reasonable alternative.

The following factors need to be considered in making the decision:
- is the patient in pain and, therefore, how quickly is intervention needed?
- how complex is the patient's medical history, and should this be managed in the practice setting, day-care setting or as an inpatient?
- has previous treatment with sedation been successful, and if so what type of sedation was used?
- can the sedation be done in the practice or does the patient need to be referred for specialist treatment?
- is an intraoral examination possible?
- are preoperative radiographs possible?
- how much treatment is required?
- what level of care is available post-treatment?
- how long are local GA waiting lists?
- what is the patient and parent/carer's preference?

Conclusions

- Many dentists will not be able to offer the full range of sedation techniques but they should be aware of local services and be able to make appropriate referrals.
- Practitioners who want to use sedation techniques with special care patients should receive training in sedation and have experience in treating medically compromised patients and those with disabilities.

- It is also essential that the whole dental team is trained in sedation and that appropriate monitoring equipment is available.
- General anaesthesia is still necessary for some special care patients and access to comprehensive dental care under GA is a service that must be maintained.

Further Reading

Boyle CA, Manley MGC and Fleming G. Sedation with oral midazolam for people with learning disabilities. Dent Update 2000;27:190-192.

Craig D, Skelly AM. Practical conscious sedation. Quintessence Publishing Co. Ltd., 2004.

Manley MCG, Skelly AM, Hamilton AG. Dental treatment for people with challenging behaviour: general anaesthesia or sedation. Br Dent J 2000;188:358-360.

Index

X

Quintessentials for General Dental Practitioners Series

in 50 volumes

Editor-in-Chief: Professor Nairn H F Wilson

The Quintessentials for General Dental Practitioners Series covers basic principles and key issues in all aspects of modern dental medicine. Each book can be read as a stand-alone volume or in conjunction with other books in the series.

Publication date, approximately

Clinical Practice, Editor: Nairn Wilson

Culturally Sensitive Oral Healthcare	available
Dental Erosion	available
Special Care Dentistry	available
Evidence Based Dentistry	Spring 2007
Dental Bleaching	Spring 2007
Infection Control for the Dental Team	Spring 2007
Therapeutics and Medical Emergencies in the Everyday Clinical Practice of Dentistry	Summer 2007

Oral Surgery and Oral Medicine, Editor: John G Meechan

Practical Dental Local Anaesthesia	available
Practical Oral Medicine	available
Practical Conscious Sedation	available
Minor Oral Surgery in Dental Practice	available

Imaging, Editor: Keith Horner

Interpreting Dental Radiographs	available
Panoramic Radiology	available
Twenty-first Century Dental Imaging	Summer 2007

Periodontology, Editor: Iain L C Chapple

Understanding Periodontal Diseases: Assessment and Diagnostic Procedures in Practice	available
Decision-Making for the Periodontal Team	available
Successful Periodontal Therapy – A Non-Surgical Approach	available
Periodontal Management of Children, Adolescents and Young Adults	available
Periodontal Medicine: A Window on the Body	available

Endodontics, Editor: John M Whitworth

Rational Root Canal Treatment in Practice	available
Managing Endodontic Failure in Practice	available
Restoring Endodontically Treated Teeth	Spring 2007

Prosthodontics, Editor: P Finbarr Allen

Teeth for Life for Older Adults	available
Complete Dentures – from Planning to Problem Solving	available
Removable Partial Dentures	available
Fixed Prosthodontics in Dental Practice	available
Occlusion: A Theoretical and Team Approach	Spring 2007
Managing Orofacial Pain in Practice	Summer 2007

Operative Dentistry, Editor: Paul A Brunton

Decision-Making in Operative Dentistry	available
Aesthetic Dentistry	available
Communicating in Dental Practice	available
Indirect Restorations	available
Choosing and Using Dental Materials	Spring 2007
Composite Restorations in Posterior Teeth	Summer 2007

Paediatric Dentistry/Orthodontics, Editor: Marie Therese Hosey

Child Taming: How to Manage Children in Dental Practice	available
Paediatric Cariology	available
Treatment Planning for the Developing Dentition	available
Managing Dental Trauma in Practice	available

General Dentistry and Practice Management, Editor: Raj Rattan

The Business of Dentistry	available
Risk Management in General Dental Practice	available
Quality Matters: From Clinical Care to Customer Service	available
Practice Management for the Dental Team	Summer 2007

Dental Team, Editor: Mabel Slater

Team Players in Dentistry	Summer 2007

Implantology, Editor: Lloyd J Searson

Implantology in General Dental Practice	available

Quintessence Publishing Co. Ltd., London